The Healing Power of Play

THE HEALING POWER OF PLAY

Working with Abused Children

ELIANA GIL, Ph.D.

THE GUILFORD PRESS

New York   *London*

Last digit is print number: 9 8 7 6 5 4 3 2

Library of Congress Cataloging-in-Publication Data

Gil, Eliana.
  The healing power of play : working with abused children /
Eliana Gil.
    p. cm.
  Includes bibliographical references and index.
  ISBN 0-89862-560-2.   ISBN 0-89862-467-3 (pbk.)
  1. Abused children—Mental health—Case studies. 2. Play
therapy—Case studies. I. Title.
  [DNLM: Child Abuse—rehabilitation—case studies. 2. Play
Therapy—in infancy & childhood—case studies. WS 320 G4632h]
RJ507.A29G55   1991
618.92′891653—dc20   ᴹ
DNLM/DLC
for Library of Congress   91-6708
                                                        CIP

To Robert Jay Green, Ph.D., who
chose me as his trainee
recognized my capacity
encouraged my intellect
tells me to reach high
always makes me laugh
allows me to feel special

Acknowledgments

Writing this book was a stressful and happy experience. While writing, I was reminded of my child clients, the traumatic events in their lives, their incredible strength and hope, and the unique ways they coped. Their courage, resiliency, and joy amaze me and inspire me.

I thank my many colleagues who inspire and stimulate me and I am greatly appreciative to my friends and family who stand by me as I tackle large and small projects. My gratitude to Toby Troffkin for her copyediting of the book, and my research assistants, David Farinella and Coco Ishi. Special thanks to my husband John, my source of strength and joy; my in-laws Norm and Eileen; my mom, Eugenia, and my brother Peter; my great kids Eric, Teresa, and Christy; my best friends, Teresa and Tony Davi, Melissa and Melinda Brown, Mary Herget, Kathy Baxter-Stern, Robert Green, Jeff Bodmer-Turner, Steve Santini, Lou Fox, Sue Scoff, my Wednesday group, and my colleagues at A STEP FORWARD.

The clinical material presented in this book is a compilation of cases. To protect the confidentiality of my clients I have changed all identifying information. Where dialogue or art work is provided, it is presented with the permission of the parents.

A portion of the first chapter of this book entitled "The Impact of Child Abuse" was adapted from the first chapter ("Behavioral Indicators of Abuse") of my book *Treatment of Adult Survivors of Childhood Abuse,* which was published in 1988. This material was adapted and reproduced with permission of Launch Press, Walnut Creek, CA.

Contents

The Healing Power of Play

The Abused Child:
Treatment Issues

THE ABUSED CHILD

Children have been subjected to differing types of maltreatment throughout history, and these atrocities are well documented (Radbill, 1980; Summit, 1988). For centuries society condoned infanticide, physical abuse, sexual abuse, and the exploitation of children's labor.

The prevalence of child maltreatment has endured throughout time and has cultivated tenacious legacies that have shaped societal response to child abuse. Those legacies include the tenet that children are the property of their parents—and expendable as well. These traditions contributed to the slow societal response in defining and responding to child abuse. In addition, society has suffered from a denial of the problem's existence and prevalence. Even the medical community, seeing the firsthand consequences of abuse in emergency rooms, reacted more slowly than one

1

might expect. In the 1940s there was some documentation of physical abuse cases appearing in hospital settings; the first article stating the possibility of parental maltreatment was written by Caffey (1946), a radiologist who cited subdural hematomas in infants who had atypical fractures of the limbs and ribs. Skepticism prevailed about the extent of this problem until 1962, when Dr. C. Henry Kempe coined the phrase "the battered child syndrome" (Kempe & Helfer, 1980) and finally succeeded in calling national attention to this persistent social problem.

Major developments have occurred since that time, the most noteworthy being the creation of laws to protect children even from their biological parents. In 1962 the first reporting law was written, and by 1964 every state had a child abuse reporting law mandating physicians to report suspected physical abuse.

The other significant evolution has been in the expansion of the definition of *child abuse*. Most states currently define child abuse in subcategories that include at least the following: physical abuse, sexual abuse, and neglect. Many states have formulated definitions that encompass psychological or emotional abuse as well as sexual exploitation, which includes child pornography and child prostitution. The list of professionals mandated to report known or suspected abuse to the authorities continues to expand.

Since the late '60s literally hundreds of research projects have focused on child abuse, particularly on child sexual abuse (Herman, 1981). A body of research has accumulated on the family dynamics of abuse, the short- and long-term effects of abuse, victim and perpetrator characteristics, and prevention and treatment strategies.

It appears that even though the empirical research is vast, studies are fraught with methodological problems due to small sample sizes and design difficulties. Finkelhor (1984) identifies a number of areas that require additional and more refined research, including the differential effects of abuse on preschoolers versus older children, the negative effects of justice system intervention, cultural differences in abuse and effects, and the differential effects by types of abuse.

Beginning with the '70s a great deal of interest has converged on the subject of sexual abuse of children, and I agree with Finkelhor (1984) that more quality research is absolutely necessary on a variety of topics of child abuse, including the differential effects of physical abuse, neglect, and emotional abuse. This information will allow clinicians to formulate more precise treatment strategies.

I will offer a brief summary of the most consistent findings in the research. It appears that the experience of parental maltreatment of children, regardless of the form it takes, has particular psychological and emotional implications for the child victim. Perhaps nowhere do we find greater evidence of this than in contemporary findings from both the research and the clinical work done with adult survivors (Briere, 1989; Courtois, 1989; Finkelhor, 1986; Gil, 1989).

MEDIATORS IN THE EFFECTS
OF CHILD ABUSE

Although findings have emerged from studies on child sexual abuse (Finkelhor, 1986; Lusk & Waterman, 1986; Wyatt & Powell, 1988), it appears that several factors mediate the impact of any type of abuse on children. These factors include the age of the child at the time of the abuse, the chronicity, the severity, the relationship to the offender, the level of threats to the child, the emotional climate of the child's family prior to the abuse, the child's mental and emotional health prior to the abuse, the amount of guilt the child feels, the sex of the victim, and the parental response to the child's victimization.

Age of the Child at the Time of Abuse

There is some discrepancy in the research on the effect of the child's age on later outcome (Adams-Tucker, 1982; Ruch & Chandler, 1982); however, a trend exists toward viewing the younger child as more vulnerable to damage. Van der Kolk (1987) states that childhood trauma is most damaging to

younger children because "uncontrollable terrifying experiences may have their most profound effects when the
central nervous system and cognitive functions have not yet
fully matured, leading to a global impairment" (p. xii).

Chronicity

There is consensus in the research that the more chronic the
abuse, the greater the impact. If the abuse continues over a
period of time, the child's sense of helplessness and vulnerability can increase, and the child has greater opportunity to utilize and refine defense mechanisms, such as
dissociation, that can become problematic later in life.

Severity

Probably the more extensive the abuse, the greater the
damage. This is obvious in cases of severe physical abuse,
which can result in physical handicaps, brain damage, and
developmental delays, and in cases of neglect, which can
result in a nonorganic failure to thrive. In sexual abuse cases
more extensive genital contact, such as penetration, has been
associated with a greater negative impact (Adams-Tucker,
1982; Mrazek, 1980).

Relationship to Offender

It is generally believed that the closer the relationship
between the offender and the child, the greater the resultant trauma (Adams-Tucker, 1982; Simari & Baskin, 1982).
The child who is abused outside the home is able to project
the badness outside the home and turn to the family for
protection and reassurance. The child abused by a loved one
learns that the person who loves him/her is also the hurtful
person.

Level of Threats

The use of threats, force, and violence also potentially wor-
sens a trauma (Ruch & Chandler, 1982). The presence of

threats may produce generalized anxiety and fear in the child. The threat need not be explicit to manipulate a child; a child can feel threatened and can feel as though he/she must keep a secret even when the threat is nonverbally communicated.

The Emotional Climate of the Child's Family

Azar and Wolfe (1989) state that "the pervasive effects on abused children's psychological and behavioral development that result from the many factors accompanying abuse in families and affecting their behavior are less understood and potentially more harmful to the children's development" (p. 452). The family dysfunction includes patterns of inter-generational abuse, inappropriate child-rearing patterns and parenting skills, social incompetence and isolation from support systems, emotional distress, inaccurate perceptions and high expectations of children, and emotional arousal and reactivity to child provocation (Wolfe, 1987). In discussing neglecting families, Polansky, Chalmers, Buttenweiser, and Williams (1979) cite generalized chaos and disorganization, matched with rampant low functioning affecting all areas of performance. Julian, Mohr, and Lapp (1980) found that the factors most often associated with incest families are family discord, mental health problems, broken family, alcohol dependence, spouse abuse, social isolation, and insufficient income. Barrett, Sykes, and Byrnes (1986) characterize incestuous families as incohesive and inflexible, with poor instrumental and affective communication and incongruent hierarchies. These types of problems create a climate where abuse can occur. Emslie and Rosenfeld (1983), in their comparison study of abused girls who were victims of incest and those who were not, concluded that the psychopathology of the girls was a consequence of severe family disorganization and no specific effects of incest could be found.

The Child's Mental and Emotional Health

If the child has good psychological health prior to the abuse, he/she is in a better position to resist the damaging effects of abuse (Adams-Tucker, 1981; Leaman, 1980). Van der Kolk (1987) asserts that "an adult with a firm sense of identity and good social support is infinitely better protected than a child, who has a lower level of cognitive development" (p. 11).

The Guilt the Child Feels

In cases of sexual abuse, it is generally agreed that if the child experiences some pleasure during sexual contact or feels somehow responsible for causing the abuse, he/she is more likely to feel guilt, which is associated with greater impact (MacFarlane & Korbin, 1983).

The Sex of the Victim

It was initially thought that males suffered less trauma than female victims (Adams-Tucker, 1982; Vander Mey & Neff, 1982); however, these beliefs were probably based on lack of knowledge about male victims. Recent research on the subject (Briere, 1989) supports earlier speculation (Finch, 1973) that male victims show long-range serious problems and greater psychopathology. Nasjleti (1980), E. Porter (1986), Risin and Koss (1987), Hunter (1990), Dimock (1988), and Lew (1988) have offered valuable insights into the impact of sexual abuse on boys and men.

Parental Responses to the Child's Victimization

Leaman (1980) and others (James & Nasjleti, 1983; Sgroi, 1982; Summit & Kryso, 1978) have repeatedly emphasized the pivotal role the nonabusive parent plays in the healing of the child. The child's recovery is greatly enhanced by a parent who believes the child and is not accusatory but is unequivocally supportive and reassuring. An unsupportive or overreactive parental response results in greater trauma (Tufts, 1984).

THE IMPACT OF CHILD ABUSE

The impact of sexual abuse more than likely can be measured along a continuum. Friedrich (1990) says:

> Sexual abuse and its impact should be seen along a continuum ranging from neutral to very negative. Sometimes when we see only one type of child or family, we may believe that abuse is either much more discrete in its impact or primarily very negative. It is important to recognize this variability because it reminds us again of the hopefulness that can be present even in traumatic events and that the possibility for positive change always exists. It also forces us to realize that there are strengths and sources of resilience in the individuals whom we see that exceed any of the curative powers that we might be able to bring to these dysfunctional systems. (p. 102)

Because children are unable to fully understand or explain the impact of abuse, professionals usually rely on the development of symptomatic behaviors to signal underlying emotional difficulties. The most common problems exhibited by child victims include affective disorders; anxiety and fear; depression; physical effects, including psychosomatic complaints, injury, and pregnancy; cognitive and school-related problems; learned helplessness; aggressive and antisocial behaviors; withdrawal; self-destructive behaviors; psychopathology; sexual problems; poor self-esteem; and problems with interpersonal relationships (Lusk & Waterman, 1986). The following categorization attempts to distinguish the most common symptomatic behaviors by type of abuse.

Sexual Abuse

Finkelhor (1986) analyzed the empirical data on short-term effects of sexual abuse and concluded that abused children regularly exhibit the following signs:

- Fear or anxiety
- Depression

- Difficulties in school
- Anger or hostility
- Inappropriate sexualized behavior
- Running away or delinquency

Physical Abuse

In a ground breaking book Martin (1976) finds that physically abused children exhibit the following:

- Impaired capacity to enjoy life
- Psychiatric symptoms, enuresis, tantrums, hyperactivity, bizarre behavior
- Low self-esteem
- Learning problems in school
- Withdrawal
- Opposition
- Hypervigilance
- Compulsivity
- Pseudomature behavior

Martin and Rodeheffer (1980) state that:

Physical abuse may result in a number of biological consequences, including death, brain damage, mental retardation, cerebral palsy, learning disabilities and sensory deficits. The neurological handicaps of physical abuse are of particular interest because of their chronicity and significance to the long-range functioning of the individual. It is estimated that between 25 and 30% of abused children who survive the attack have brain damage or neurological dysfunction resulting directly from physical trauma about the head. (p. 207)

Martin and Rodeheffer also quote a study conducted by the National Center for Prevention of Child Abuse and Neglect in Denver in 1976 that found that physically abused children have deficits in gross motor development, speech, and language. They go on to say that physically abused children exhibit the following:

Interpersonal ambivalence

Hypervigilant preoccupation with the behavior of others

Constant mobilization of defenses in anticipation of danger

Inability to perceive and act on the environment in pursuit of mastery

Impaired socialization skills with peers

Frustration from inability to meet expectations of others

Defensiveness in social contacts

"Chameleon nature" (shifting behavior to accommodate to others)

Learned helplessness ("To try a task and fail is more dangerous than not to try at all")

Tendency to care for their parents physically and emotionally

Lack of object permanence or object constancy (distortion of normal object relations)

Reidy (1982), summarizing traits of physically abused children, found that they exhibit aggression and hatred, uncontrollable negativistic behavior and severe temper tantrums, lack of impulse control, emotionally disturbed behavior both at home and at school, and withdrawn or inhibited behavior. Reidy in his own study (1982) finds that abused children (1) express significantly more fantasy aggression on the Thematic Apperception Test (TAT) than other children; (2) exhibit aggressive behavior more frequently than other children; and (3) express significantly more fantasy aggression in their natural homes than they do in foster homes.

Kent (1980) finds that physically abused children (1) tend to have more problems managing aggressive behavior than other children, and (2) tend to have more problems establishing peer relationships than other children.

Martin (1976) makes an important point:

The child's personality is affected and shaped by the total environment in which [the child] lives. The specific incidents of physical assault are a psychic trauma. However, the broader picture, which may include rejection, chaos, deprivation, distorted parental perceptions, unrealistic expectations as well as hospitalization, separation, foster placement and frequent home changes, is in the long run more significant to the child's development. (p. 107)

Neglect

The dynamics of child neglect differ significantly from the dynamics of physical and sexual abuse. The greatest single difference is that physically and sexually abused children receive attention from their parents. The attention is inappropriate, excessive, harsh, and damaging, but the parent is definitely *aware* of the child's existence. Energy is directed toward the child. Neglectful parents do the opposite; overwhelmed, lethargic, and incapacitated, they feel or express little interest in the child. They *withhold attention;* they do not stimulate the child; they rarely make physical or emotional contact. In extreme cases the neglectful parent seems to be unaware that the child exists.

Polansky et al. (1981) finds that neglected children exhibit the following:

- "Deprivation–detachment"
- Massive repression of feelings (affect inhibition)
- Impaired ability to empathize with others
- Violence
- Delinquency
- Decrease in general intellectual ability (due to lack of cognitive stimulation on the part of the parent)

Kent (1980) also finds developmental delays in neglected children.

Emotional Abuse

Garbarino, Guttmann, and Seeley (1986) describe emotionally abused children as "showing evidence of psychosocial harm," as evidenced by the following signs and symptoms:

- Behavioral problems (anxiety, aggression, hostility)
- Emotional disturbance (feelings of being unloved, unwanted, unworthy)
- Inappropriate social disturbance (negative view of the world)
- In infants, irritability and, in some cases, nonorganic failure to thrive
- Anxious attachment to parents
- Fear or distrust
- Low self-esteem
- Feelings of inferiority; withdrawal; lack of communication
- Self-destructive behavior (self-mutilation, depression, suicidal tendencies)
- Tendency to act as caretaker to parents
- Delinquency or truancy

Garbarino et al. summarizes their findings:

> The psychologically maltreated child is often identified by personal characteristics, perceptions, and behaviors that convey low self-esteem, a negative view of the world, and internalized or externalized anxieties and aggressions. Whether the child clings to adults or avoids them, his or her social behavior and responses are inappropriate and exceptional. (p. 63)

It should be noted that some victims of child abuse seem to emerge unscathed. Garbarino et al. discuss "stress-resistant" children who become prosocial and competent in spite of their harsh, or even hostile, upbringing. He concludes that these children receive "compensatory doses of psychological nurturance and sustenance [that] enable them to develop social competence, that fortify self-esteem, and [that] offer a positive social definition of self" (p. 9).

Anthony and Cohler (1987), in their extensive studies of resiliency, conclude:

> The child shares with other organisms a biological tendency to achieve wholeness—not as a static state, but as a

dynamic, flexible balance that permits recoil or regression and rebound of progress. Biological rhythms of activity and rest provide a basic pattern for acceptance of restitution from the outside. The whole range of resources may be involved: biochemical factors, including hormones and endorphins; the interaction of cortical, subcortical, autonomic nervous system, and glandular activity; and psychological forces. All these resources interact, mobilizing regenerative power. Residues of experiences of resilience after physical or emotional disturbance contribute both a sense of "feeling good" and also a consolidation of confidence, optimism, and ability to respond to or seek help when faced with threats in the future. The drive toward integration, then, utilizes selective combinations of other drives and capacities available at a given stage of the child's development. (p. 101)

In the following section I offer some clinical observations based on my own experience in providing therapy to abused children. I do not attempt to categorize behavioral indicators by type of abuse because they frequently overlap.

CLINICAL OBSERVATIONS

The problem behaviors of abused children are manifested internally or externally. The behaviors described in the following paragraphs are ones that are regularly observed by me and by those of my colleagues who specialize in the treatment of abused children. I consider them to be indicators of abuse. However, these (and those already listed) are not *conclusive* of abuse in and of themselves. Children who are not abused but who live in dysfunctional families or suffer crises such as divorce or parental death may also exhibit these behaviors.

Internalized Behavior

Children who exhibit internalized behavior tend to be isolated and withdrawn. They attempt to negotiate the abuse by themselves; they do not interact with others. These children frequently

Appear withdrawn and unmotivated to seek interactions
Exhibit clinical signs of depression
Lack spontaneity and playfulness
Are overcompliant
Develop phobias with unspecified precipitants
Appear hypervigilant and anxious
Experience sleep disorders or night terrors
Demonstrate regressed behavior
Have somatic complaints (headaches, stomachaches)
Develop eating disorders
Engage in substance and drug abuse
Make suicide gestures
Engage in self-mutilation[1]
Dissociate

Externalized Behavior

Conversely, children with externalized manifestations
engage in behavior directed toward others; they exhibit out-
ward expression of their emotions. Such children are aggressive, hostile, and destructive; provocative (eliciting abuse);
violent, sometimes killing or torturing animals[2]; prone to
destructive behaviors including fire-setting; and sexualized.

---

[1]Self-mutilation must be distinguished from suicide gesturing. Self-mutilation
seems to be utilized for a variety of reasons, including grounding (from dissociative or depressed states), comforting (especially when children have been
physically abused and believe love and pain go together), satisfaction of need
for parental care (as when foster children miss their parents and cannot see
them). Finally, some children use self-mutilation to ascertain their own
humanity. Self-mutilation is usually found in adolescents; however, younger
abused children can begin to develop the more typical ritualistic, hidden
behaviors associated with older children and adults. If left uninterrupted, this
coping mechanism can continue well into adulthood. Numerous adult clients
have stated this to be the case.

[2]The killing and torturing of animals is a significant cry for help; these children
are in grievous distress. Two common clinical findings to explain this behavior
are the following: (1) the child is behaviorally reenacting his/her own abuse on
a smaller victim and (2) the child is rehearsing suicide. The stronger the child's
emotional attachment to the animal, the more alarming this behavior is.

They are often more readily identified because their behavior creates a problem for other people.

Internalized and externalized behaviors can overlap; children can have differing types of reactions to any specific feeling. Fear, for example, has been observed to have three types of reaction to perceived threat: (1) motor reactions, such as avoidance, escape, and tentative approach; (2) subjective reactions, such as verbal reports of discomfort, distress, and terror; and (3) physiological reactions, such as heart palpitations, profuse sweating, and rapid breathing (Barrios & O'Dell, 1989, p.168). In my experience, a child may present with internalized behaviors and develop or exhibit externalized behaviors during treatment. My hypothesis is that as these children learn to trust the therapist and are encouraged to express their hidden emotions, they become more able to show feelings such as anger and hostility.

Special Issues

Abused children can also develop two special behaviors: dissociation and sexualization. Both are important to assess and treat and seem to be frequently misunderstood, remaining undiagnosed and untreated.

Dissociative Phenomena

The *Diagnostic and Statistical Manual of Mental Disorders* defines dissociative phenomena as "a disturbance or alteration in the normally integrative functions of identity, memory, or consciousness" (1987, p. 269). The DSM-III-R categorizes three types of dissociative phenomena: (1) multiple personality disorder (disturbance in identity), (2) depersonalization disorder (disturbance in identity), and (3) psychogenic amnesia or fugue (disturbance in memory). Dissociative phenomena may be represented along a continuum, with multiple personality disorder, the most extreme form of dissociation, occurring at the endpoint. Emerging empirical data reveal an indisputable correlation between early severe childhood abuse and multiple personality disorder (Kluft,

1985; Putnam, 1989). Multiplicity is believed to begin in childhood, yet diagnosis usually occurs much later. Historically, there has been a speedier identification of dissociation and multiplicity in adults. Clinicians working with severely abused children are well advised to research the area of childhood multiplicity (Kluft, 1985; Peterson, 1990).

Dissociative phenomena are *clearly linked to trauma.* According to Eth and Pynoos (1985), psychic trauma occurs "when an individual is exposed to an overwhelming event resulting in helplessness in the face of intolerable danger, anxiety, and instinctual arousal" (p. 38). Clearly, abuse is a psychic trauma to children, the more so by virtue of their size, dependency, and vulnerability.

Sexualized Behavior

Finkelhor (1986) has developed a four-factor conceptual model for understanding the "traumagenic dynamics" occurring in sexual abuse. The four factors are *traumatic sexualization, stigmatization, powerlessness, and betrayal,* each with its respective dynamics, psychological impact, and behavioral manifestations (see Table 1.1). Finkelhor and Browne (1985) define traumatic sexualization as "a process in which a child's sexuality [including both sexual feelings and sexual attitudes] is shaped in a developmentally inappropriate and interpersonally dysfunctional fashion as the result of sexual abuse (p. 531). Finkelhor (1986, pp. 186–187) provides information conceptualizing the sexualization of child victims (see Table 1.1).

My own clinical observations of sexually abused children are consistent with Finkelhor's concept of traumatic sexualization as well as with the conclusions of Johnson-Cavanaugh's (1988) and Friedrich's (1988) pioneering efforts in this area. Sexually abused children develop an excessive and abnormal interest in sex, an interest that is frequently expressed in precocious sexual activity. One of the difficulties that arise in assessing children's sexual behaviors is the scarcity of contemporary normative data on the development of children's sexuality. Sgroi, Bunk, and Wabrek (1988) have

TABLE 1.1. Traumatic Sexualization

Dynamics
Child rewarded for sexual behavior inappropriate to developmental
   level
Offender exchanges attention and affection for sex
Sexual parts of child fetishized
Offender transmits misconceptions about sexual behavior and
   morality
Conditioning of sexual activity with negative memories and emotions

Psychological impact
Increased salience of sexual issues
Confusion about sexual identity
Confusion about sexual norms
Confusion of sex with love and care getting or care giving
Negative associations to sexual activities and arousal sensations
Aversion to sex or intimacy

Behavioral manifestations
Sexual preoccupations and compulsive sexual behaviors
Precocious sexual activity
Aggressive sexual behaviors
Promiscuity
Prostitution
Sexual dysfunctions

---

combined their clinical experience working with normal and
troubled children to offer a developmental framework for
children's sexuality. I have found this framework (presented
in Table 1.2) helpful in determining whether a child's sexual
behavior indicates a need to intervene.

Berliner, Manaois, and Monastersky (1986) concur that
pathological sexual behaviors in children are distinguishable
from developmentally appropriate sexual play. In their
model, they see disturbances along dimensions of severity.
The most severe type of sexualized behavior is coercive,
including the use of physical force and resultant injury.
Berliner and associates describe another dimension as consisting of developmentally precocious behavior that includes
attempted or completed intercourse without coercion. Lastly,
they list sexual behaviors considered inappropriate, which

TABLE 1.2. Children's Sexuality

Age range	Patterns of activity	Sexual behaviors
Preschool (0–5 years)	Intense curiosity; taking advantage of opportunities to explore the universe	Masturbation; looking at others' bodies
Primary school (6–10 years)	Game playing with peers and with younger children; creating opportunities to explore the universe	Masturbation; looking at others' bodies; sexual exposure of self to others; sexual fondling of peers or younger children in play or game-like atmosphere
Preadolescence (10–12 years); adolescence (13–18 years)	Individuation; separation from family; distancing from parents; developing relationships with peers; practicing intimacy with peers of both sexes; "falling in love"	Masturbation; sexual exposure; voyeurism; open-mouth kissing; sexual fondling; simulated intercourse; sexual penetration behaviors and intercourse

can include persistent, public masturbation that can cause pain or irritation; touching or asking to touch others' genitals; excessive interest in sexual matters, reflected in play, art, or conversation; and sexually stylized behavior imitative of adult sexual relationships.

As the framework of Sgroi and associates, as well as of Berliner and her colleagues, clearly illustrates, children's sexual behaviors tend to *progress* over time, with extreme behavior being indicative of psychological disturbance. Premature sexual activity in children always suggests two possible stimulants: experience and exposure. The child exhibiting premature sexual activity may have experienced sexual contact with an adult or older child and may be mimicking the learned behavior, or the child may have been overstimulated by exposure to explicit sexual activity and may be acting this activity out. Many young children have access to soft- or hard-core pornography on their television sets.

An additional characteristic of many sexualized children is a disinhibition of masturbatory behavior. A child who has not been sexually abused will abruptly stop masturbating when someone enters the room; sexually abused children, possibly having learned the sexual behavior with another person, may continue to masturbate.

Clinicians have reported sophisticated and focused sexual behavior on the part of sexually abused children. This behavior is always unusual and alarming. These children may enter a room, remove their underwear, and masturbate, hump, or attempt to engage the clinician in sexual activity. This is understandable; they have been conditioned to behave this way. Nevertheless, the behavior must be extinguished for a variety of reasons. The child can literally become a threat to younger (or older) children and may request or force sexual contact. It is possible that the child will approach someone who will be unable or unwilling to set the appropriate limits; the child then becomes a potential victim again. In addition, the more extreme masturbatory behavior can cause injuries and infections that require medical attention. Lastly, a child who behaves in these inappropriate and potentially dangerous ways will elicit a negative response from others and be singled out for rejection.

The therapist must therefore set and speedily enforce consistent and directive limits on the child and must suggest alternative behaviors. These interventions must be shared with parents and caretakers to maintain a consistent response. The therapist might, for example, say, "It's not OK for you to touch private parts of my body or to kiss my mouth" or "It's not OK for you to take off your underwear in my office." These limits must be followed immediately by the suggestion of an alternative behavior: "I can see you're trying to get my attention; to do that, you can touch my hand and call my name" or "I can see you're trying to show me how you feel. To do that, you can draw me a picture, write me a card, tell me a story, or talk to me about your feelings."

Behavioral symptoms reveal the child's distress; they are red flags that indicate underlying concerns in the child. The symptomatic behavior usually draws attention to the child; parents, school personnel, or others may seek counseling for the child upon noticing the inappropriate behaviors. However, while symptomatic behaviors may respond promptly to treatment, the underlying issues frequently require additional care.

THE IMPACT OF TRAUMA

Many victimized children may also be traumatized. While the two terms are often used interchangeably, their meanings are quite distinct. Victimization has evolved into a concept with broad-based application. A person may report feeling victimized by a strenuous job interview, a rigorous exam, or a demanding funding source; minority groups often feel victimized by policies or attitudes of the majority group; students have stated their perception of themselves as victims of a male-dominated administration. A person can be victimized without being traumatized. A person who experiences trauma, however, will always be victimized during the traumatic event.

In addition to treating such victimization issues as those delineated by Herman (1981), Kempe and Kempe (1984), Martin (1976), and Sgroi (1982), it becomes critical, when treating child victims of abuse, to assess the diverse impact of trauma, as described by Eth and Pynoos (1985), Kluft (1985), Putnam (1989), and van der Kolk (1987). The clinician then devises a therapeutic motif that encompasses a response to both victimization and traumatization issues.

As mentioned previously, Eth and Pynoos (1985) believe that a psychic trauma occurs "when an individual is exposed to an overwhelming event resulting in helplessness in the face of intolerable danger, anxiety, and instinctual arousal" (p. 38). Van der Kolk (1987) notes that the trauma response is affected by numerous factors, including the severity of the assault and the genetic predisposition, developmental phase, social support, prior trauma, and preexisting personality of the child. Of special importance is van der Kolk's belief that children are at greater risk for traumatic effects because they do not have an established identity and their repertoire of coping behaviors is limited.

Freud initially regarded psychiatric problems as manifestations of early childhood traumas, interpreting the cognitive, emotional, and behavioral symptoms of hysterical patients as symbolic repetitions of early traumatic events. He saw these repetitions as attempts to release excess energy and gain mastery. When Freud withdrew these ideas in favor of the notion of childhood fantasies, and "misperceptions of actual events," the psychoanalytic interest in trauma was temporarily lost.

In the last two decades, there has been a resurgence of interest in the consequences of specific traumas. Van der Kolk (1987) points out that while effects of specific traumas such as war, concentration camps, and rape are described as separate entities, closer examination makes it clear that "the human response to overwhelming and uncontrollable life events is remarkably consistent although the nature of the trauma, the age of the victim, predisposing personality, and community response all have an important effect on ultimate posttraumatic adaptation" (p. 2). He goes on to state that the core features of the posttraumatic syndrome are fairly consistent. Thus, it becomes evident that many of the psychological consequences of child abuse can be considered posttraumatic reenactments of unresolved trauma. Eth and Pynoos (1985) believe that "children's early responses to psychic trauma generally involve deleterious effects on cognition (including memory, school performance, and learning), affect, interpersonal relations, impulse control and behavior, vegetative function, and the formation of symptoms" (p. 41). Wolfenstein (1965) states that young traumatized children feel the most helpless and passive and require the most assistance from the outside in order to reestablish psychic equilibrium.

Terr (1990) asserts that "traumatized children repeat in

actions. Whereas adults who are shocked or severely stressed tend to talk about it, dream, or to visualize, children take far more action" (p. 265). Terr also states that even though traumatic events are external, they "quickly become incorporated into the mind," particularly when the individual feels "utter helplessness" during the traumatic events (p. 8). Others (Bergen, 1958; Eth & Pynoos, 1985; Maclean, 1977) have observed the way preschool abused children engage in play reenactment of the trauma. Wallerstein and Kelly (1975) describe the posttraumatic play as "burdened, constricted, and joyless."

Earlier I indicated that central to the treatment of adult survivors is the assessment of trauma resolution. Trauma can be resolved in positive, negative, and functional ways. Positive resolution occurs when

> the adult is able to process the trauma in a realistic way, experiencing whatever levels of pain, anger, or loss are elicited by a clear memory of the event,.....perceives the event accurately, and does not feel irrationally responsible for having caused it....[The adult] is able to understand that the experience occurred in the past, and no longer feels devastated by the memory of the event, as if it were a clear and recurring danger in the present...The person does not feel compelled to repeat the event, either consciously or unconsciously. (Gil, 1989, p. 114)

People who achieve this type of resolution break previous patterns of helplessness and feel more in control of their lives. The trauma no longer dominates their mental life.

A negative trauma resolution is in direct contrast to positive resolution and is destructive and constrictive to the individual. The person continues to live in the emotional environment of the traumatic event. Kardiner (1941) recognizes five features of human response to trauma:

- Persistence of a startle response and irritability
- Proclivity to explosive outbursts of anger
- Fixation on trauma

- Constriction of general level of personality functioning
- Atypical dream life

When the individual has a negative trauma resolution, these symptoms persist and are exacerbated by stress. Most typical of the negative effects of unresolved trauma are feelings both of reliving the trauma through intrusive thoughts or dreams and of numbing. These responses are now understood to be psychologically and physiologically based. (The diagnostic category Post-traumatic Stress Disorder [PTSD] was incorporated into the DSM-III-R in 1980.) Many individuals with unresolved trauma have symptoms of PTSD and seek counseling for relief of these symptoms, which include nightmares, intrusive flashbacks, emotionality, physical sensations, and auditory hallucinations. Most clinicians who have experience working with victims of trauma agree that the traumatic event must eventually be brought into awareness and put into perspective or the intrusion will persist (Figley, 1985).

A functional trauma resolution is one that works on a temporary basis but cannot be sustained over time. When operative, such a resolution successfully avoids uncomfortable stimuli and relies on defenses such as denial and suppression. However, external circumstances may render the resolution ineffective, catapulting the survivor into a crisis.

As stated earlier, dissociation is strongly correlated with trauma. This connection was recognized very early: Briquet first formulated the concept of dissociation in 1859, and Janet (1889) first pointed out that dissociated states often follow childhood sexual or physical abuse. Dissociation is understood as a process of separating, segregating, and isolating chunks of information, perceptions, memories, motivations, and affects. Dissociation serves as a defense against severe stress, allowing the individual to protect against the original trauma but leaving a predisposition to react to subsequent stress or familiar stimuli as if they were a reoccurrence of the trauma. It is remarkable to observe adult survivors of abuse experience affective and physiologic reactions without knowing the original trauma in their history.

Clinicians seeking to help abuse victims must become conversant with the treatment of dissociation, since it is such a common feature for trauma survivors. Braun (1988), describes his BASK model, explaining that the main stream of consciousness is made up of four processes—Behavior, Affect, Sensation, and Knowledge—functioning along a time continuum. When the integral BASK components are consistently congruent over time, consciousness is stable and the mental processes are healthy. Braun asserts that "the goal of psychotherapy is to obtain congruence across the BASK dimensions in space/time, thus yielding a decrease of dissociated thought processes, a decreased need for the defense of dissociation, and more control over interactions with the environment" (p. 23).

Working with traumatized children affords us an incredible opportunity to address the trauma shortly after its occurrence and prior to the strengthening of defensive mechanisms.

Of particular interest is the concept that unresolved traumas will leak into consciousness through dreams, memories, sensations, and behavioral reenactments. These events can be seen as the psyche's attempt to uncover the trauma and discharge the accompanying feelings, which were previously constricted in an attempt to postpone or avoid emotional discomfort.

Provided with a safe and supportive environment, children, closer to the source of their trauma, may generate a distinctive type of play that indicates prior trauma. Terr (1990) declares that traumatized children "appear to have two behavioral options, to play or to reenact" (p. 265). She goes on to say that this type of posttraumatic play is very distinctive. Terr first observed this play during her work with 23 schoolchildren who had been kidnapped and buried in a bus in Chowchilla, California. All the children returned home safely and afforded Dr. Terr the opportunity to conduct a longitudinal study on victims of trauma (in process). Terr (1983) has defined 11 aspects of posttraumatic play:

> Compulsive repetition; unconscious link between the play and the traumatic event; literalness of play with simple defenses only; failure to relieve anxiety; wide age range; varying lag time prior to its development; carrying power to nontraumatized youngsters; contagion to new generations of children; danger; use of doodling, talking, typing, and audio duplication as modes of repeated play; and possibility of therapeutically retracing posttraumatic play to an earlier trauma. (p. 309)

Terr (1983) states that it is very unusual to directly observe posttraumatic play in the office, probably due to the secretive nature of the play. However, in my experience, *setting a context for trauma work* can facilitate the child's posttraumatic play or behavioral re-enactments. It appears that through this type of play we can assist the child toward trauma resolution. Johnson (1989) notes that the central tasks of posttrauma treatment include "reexperience, release, and reorganization" (p. 119). The child who is unable to relieve anxiety or move beyond the literal scenario that has been recreated may benefit from the clinician's participation in the posttraumatic play. Techniques for setting the context and suggested interventions during the play will be discussed later in this volume and demonstrated in the case vignettes.

In Terr's subsequent work (1990) she cautions that posttraumatic play can fail to relieve the child's anxiety and, in fact, "if the child reenacts often enough, his developing character will be affected, leading to 'maladaptive character structures'" (p. 269). Terr emphatically states that "fixing these character realignments following traumatic maladjustments is probably the most significant contribution a psychiatrist can make to the traumatized child's future" (p. 270). Posttraumatic play, according to Terr, can be "dangerous," since "posttraumatic play may create more terror than was consciously there when the game started" (p. 239). She regards posttraumatic play as resistant to interpretations or clarifications but adds that behavioral interventions may render effective results. This information highlights the need to teach parents and child victims alike the strategies for coping with fear and anxiety.

The clinician who chooses to work with abused and traumatized children is advised to establish a method for assessing the need for trauma resolution work, providing context and direction, facilitating posttraumatic play, and making timely interventions. This cannot be done without a thorough understanding of trauma and its impact. The clinician also encounters few rules or guidelines, because studies focusing on treatment outcomes of work with abused children are "almost nonexistent" in the literature (Azar & Wolfe, 1989, p. 481).

The Child Therapies:
Application in Work
with Abused Children

Closer than the moon, even closer than the
depths of the seas,
the minds of children seem to most people
not only mysterious,
but impenetrable.
—J. ALEXIS BURLAND & THEODORE B. COHEN

Child therapy is described by Sours (1980) as "a relationship between the child and the therapist, aimed primarily at symptom resolution and attaining adaptive stability" (p. 275). Child therapy, as a separate and distinct type of work, has been evolving since 1909, when Freud first attempted psychotherapy with the now historic patient Little Hans. The term *child therapy* is often used interchangeably with the term *play therapy* although play was not used directly in the therapy of children until 1920 when Hermine Hug-Hellmuth began using play for the diagnosis and treatment of childhood emotional problems (Schaefer, 1980). Melanie Klein and Anna Freud formulated the theory and practice of psychoanalytic play therapy some 10 years later.

While most child therapists agree that play is the most effective medium for conducting therapy with children, others (Freiberg, 1965; Sandler, Kennedy, & Tyson, 1980) have raised questions as to whether play produces structural change, have pointed to the nebulous quality of play, and have dismissed it as consisting of neither dream material nor free association. Schaeffer (1983) contends that "it is somewhat difficult for anyone interested in play and play therapy to gain a clear understanding of what is meant by the term play because no single, comprehensive definition of the term has been developed" (p. 2). However, the potential benefits of play are well documented. In his literature review Schaeffer found descriptions of play as "pleasurable," "intrinsically complete," "independent from external rewards or other people," "noninstrumental, with no goal," and "not occurring in novel or frightening situations." Schaeffer suggests that play is person- rather than object-dominated.

Schaeffer (1980) further asserts that "one of the most firmly established principles of psychology is that play is a process of development for a child" (p. 95). Play has been alternately depicted as a mechanism for developing "problem-solving and competence skills" (White, 1966); a process that allows children to "mentally digest" experiences and situations (Piaget, 1969); an "emotional laboratory" in which the child learns to cope with his/her environment (Erikson, 1963); a way that the child talks, with "toys as his words" (Ginott, 1961); and a way to deal with behaviors and concerns through "playing it out" (Erikson, 1963). Nickerson (1973) views play activities as the main therapeutic approach for children because it is a natural medium for self-expression, facilitates a child's communication, allows for a cathartic release of feelings, can be renewing and constructive, and allows the adult a window to observe the child's world. Nickerson points out that the child feels at home in a play setting, readily relates to toys, and will play out concerns

with them. Chethik (1989) makes an important point about
the use of play as therapy: "Play in itself will not ordinarily
produce changes...the therapist's interventions and utiliza-
tions of the play are critical" (p. 49). In addition, the clinician
must serve as a participant–observer, rather than a
playmate. I believe that play in therapy must be facilitated
by an involved clinician in a meaningful way. Some of the
most frequent errors made in child therapy are allowing a
child to play randomly over an extended period of time,
ignoring the child's play, and providing the kind of toys that
do not promote self-expression.

As interest in child therapy has grown and as the number of child-specific referrals has increased, a variety of
therapeutic techniques, games, and toys have also evolved.
Play therapy has blossomed into a multifaceted and exciting
field of study.

THE HISTORICAL DEVELOPMENT OF PLAY THERAPY

As mentioned earlier, Sigmund Freud in 1909 was the first
to use play to uncover his client's unconscious fears and
concerns. Hermine Hug-Hellmuth began using play as a part
of her treatment of children in 1920 (Hug-Hellmuth, 1921)
and 10 years later, Melanie Klein and Anna Freud formulated the theory and practice of psychoanalytic play therapy.
This type of play therapy continues to be one of the most
respected forms of child therapy, usually conducted by
analysts.

Psychoanalytic Play Therapy

Anna Freud and Melanie Klein wrote extensively about how
they incorporated play into their psychoanalytic technique.
Whereas the former advocated using play mainly to build a
strong positive relationship between child and therapist,
the latter proposed using it as a direct substitute for ver-

balizations. The primary goal of their approach was "to help children work through difficulties or trauma by helping them gain insight" (Schaefer & O'Connor, 1983). Anna Freud has repeatedly pointed out that "the essential task [of therapy] is to remove the obstacles that impede [the child's] development and to allow his progressive developmental forces and ego resources to complete the task of development" (Nagera, 1980, p. 22). Klein (1937) felt that an analysis of the child's transference relationship with the therapist was the main source of insight into the child's underlying conflict.

Freud and Klein took the basic concept of free association, one of the basic precepts of adult analysis, and in its place substituted the child's natural tendency to play (Nagera, 1980). They proposed that play uncovered the child's unconscious conflicts and desires and that play was the child's way of free-associating. While Klein proposed that the child's play is "fully equivalent" to the adult's free associations and "equally available for interpretation," Freud's theory viewed play not as an equivalent to adult free associations but as an ego-mediated mode of behavior "yielding a substantial body of data" but requiring supplementation from a variety of sources, including parents (Esman, 1983). Psychoanalytic play therapy, predicated on the analysis of resistance and transference, emphasizes the use of interpretation, recognizing the child's ability to use play symbolically to manifest internal concerns. Nagera (1980) documents that even though significant differences existed in the theoretical tenets of Freud and Klein in the beginning, throughout the years there has been more of a convergence between the two theories. Fries (1937), a student of Anna Freud's, delineates the distinctions between the two theories, emphasizing Freud's preference to withhold interpretation.

Esman (1983) describes the focus of play in psychoanalytic child therapy: "It allows for the communication of wishes, fantasies, and conflicts in ways the child can tolerate affectively and express at the level of his or her cognitive capacities" (p. 19). He goes on to say that the therapist's function is to "observe, attempt to understand, integrate, and ultimately communicate the meanings of the child's play in order to promote the child's understanding of his or her conflict toward the end of more adaptive resolution" (p. 19).

Structured Play Therapies

In the late 1930s, a more goal-oriented therapy, known as "structured therapy," was developed. This therapy emerged from a psychoanalytic framework and from a belief in the cathartic value of play and the active role of the therapist in determining the course and focus of therapy (Schaefer & O'Connor, 1983).

Anna Freud had initially found the use of affective release useful, but on the basis of later experience she encouraged this type of work only in cases of severe traumatic neuroses. David Levy (1939), stimulated by Anna Freud's conclusion and by Sigmund Freud's concept of "repetition compulsion," introduced the concept of "release therapy" for children who had experienced trauma. Levy helped the child recreate the traumatic event through play. The goal of this type of play was to help the child assimilate the negative thoughts and feelings associated with the trauma by reenacting it over and over again. Levy cautioned against using this technique too early in therapy, before a strong therapeutic relationship had been formed. In addition, he took care to avoid "flooding," in which the child is overcome by strong emotions and thus unable to assimilate them.

Other well-known contributors to the literature on structured therapies include Hambidge and Solomon. Solomon (1938) thought that helping a child express rage and fear through play without experiencing the feared negative consequences would have an abreactive effect. Hambidge (1955) was even more directive than Levy, who provided toys to facilitate the child's recreation of the trauma: Hambidge facilitated the child's abreaction by *directly* recreating the event or life situation in play.

Relationship Therapies

Otto Rank and Carl Rogers, also considered *non-directive* therapists, were the major proponents of relationship therapy, which is based on a particular theory of personality "which assumes that an individual has within himself not only the ability to solve his own problems but also a growth force that makes mature behavior more satisfying than immature behavior" (Schaefer, 1980, p. 101). This type of therapy promotes the full acceptance of the child as he/she is, and stresses the importance of the therapeutic relationship. Moustakas (1966), another prominent leader in the field of child therapy, emphasizes the genuineness of the therapist as pivotal to the success of therapy. He strongly advocates the importance of the here-and-now as the nucleus of therapeutic success. Axline (1969) also gives credence to the importance of the therapeutic relationship, viewing it as the "deciding factor" (p. 74). Axline's writings, particularly the widely touted book *Dibbs in Search of Self* (1964), have clearly delineated the benefits and desirability of nondirective therapy.

Behavior Therapies

In the 1960s the behavior therapies, based on the principles of learning theory were developed. Such therapies apply the concepts of reinforcement and modeling to relieve behavior problems in children. The behavioral approaches are precisely concerned with the problem behavior itself, not with the past or with feelings that might have preceded or accompanied the behaviors. No attempts are made to achieve affective release, to do cathartic or abreactive work, or to help children express feelings. Behavioral approaches are applied directly to children in the playroom or are taught to parents for use in the home. This type of therapy has broad application to childhood problems, particularly those that stem from a lack of adult guidance and limit setting. Within this framework play is used as a means to an end, not as inherently valuable in and of itself.

Group Therapy

Slavson (1947) experimented with group situations in 1947, guiding latency-age children through activities, games, and arts and crafts designed to help them "release emotional and physical tensions" (p. 101). In 1950, Schiffer developed what began to be known as "therapeutic play groups" (Rothenberg & Schiffer, 1966) in which children could interact freely with minimal intervention from the clinicians. The unique aspect of this type of therapy, according to Schaefer (1980), is that "the child has to learn to share an adult with other children" (p. 101). Group therapy enjoys a certain contemporary popularity, partly because it can be provided at lower cost and partly because there has been a growing belief in the effectiveness of this modality. Yalom (1975) documents numerous "curative" benefits provided by group therapy, including the following: installation of hope, universality, imparting of information, altruism, corrective recapitulation of the primary family group, development of socializing techniques, imitative behavior, interpersonal learning, group cohesiveness, catharsis, and existential factors. Kraft (1980) elucidates that effective group treatment must contain the following elements:

> Leadership, preferably with male and female co-therapists, involves developing cohesiveness, identifying goals for the group, showing the group how to function, keeping the group task-oriented, serving as a model, and representing a value system. In carrying out these tasks, the leader may offer clarification of reality, analysis of transactions, brief educational input, empathic statements acknowledging his own feelings and those of members, and at times delineating the feeling states at hand in the group. (p. 129)

Group therapy has traditionally been believed to have application to the treatment of abusive parents (Kempe & Helfer, 1980). A treatment approach used effectively with abusive parents is known as Parents Anonymous (PA), founded in California in 1970. PA uses a formerly abusive parent as a group facilitator in addition to the mental health professional. There are currently over 1,200 PA groups in the United States.

Another very well-known treatment model, Parents United, relies heavily on the group format. Parents United was established in 1975 by Dr. Hank Giarretto as the self-help component of the Child Sexual Abuse Treatment Program (Giarretto, Giarretto, & Sgroi, 1984), now known as the Community as Extended Family. Separate groups are formed for the incestuous parents and for the non-abusive partners. The children's groups are known as Daughters and Sons United, and the groups for adult survivors are known as Adults Molested as Children (AMAC) groups. There are currently over 135 active Parents United programs across the United States.

Mandell, Damon, et al. (1989) wrote a useful and timely book on group treatment for abused children, with parallel treatment for caretakers. Throughout the book the authors use different play techniques to help the children open up about their abuse and to build trust among themselves. They defined the objectives of group treatment as follows:

- Define acceptable behavior of group members and introduce a respect for boundaries.
- Promote group interaction and reinforce cooperative efforts.
- Introduce and encourage the discussion of common experiences to reinforce a feeling of togetherness and promote group cohesion for both children and caretakers.
- Improve self-esteem through validation of individual feelings and ideas, acknowledging each member's importance in contributing to the group experience.
- Help group members to understand the purpose of the group.
- Enhance caretakers' capacity to begin to view their children with increased sensitivity, understanding and empathy. (p. 27)

Another pilot project, by Corder, Haizlip, and DeBoer (1990), used structured group therapy to treat sexually abused children ages 6 to 8, and focused on issues comparable to those of Mandell and associates. The goals in the pilot project included integrating the trauma, improving self-esteem, improving problem-solving skills, self-protection for the future, improving ability to seek help, and enhancement of the child's relationship to the nonabusive parent.

In another preliminary group project with sexually abused boys, Friedrich, Berliner, Urquiza, and Beilke (1990) advocate more open-ended therapy and selection of group members by developmental level (not chronological age) in order to promote better peer interaction.

Group therapy is not without its controversy. I have often heard the concern that the group might inadvertently encourage the child to overidentify with the victim role and that groups have the potential of "contaminating" one child with the emotional concerns of another. Yet another concern, which I share, is that sometimes groups are run in random ways, go on for indefinite periods of time, lack clear goals, and suffer from inconsistent and inexperienced leadership. However, these concerns are discussed in the book by Mandell and associates and do not undermine the potential benefits of the group experience.

Sand Tray Therapy

No summary of the major models of child therapy would be complete without making note of the significant contribution of Dora Kalff (1980), who created sand therapy. Sand therapy, based on the principles of Jungian therapy, sees the sand tray as symbolic of the child's psyche. The sand therapist interprets the child's use of symbols and placement of objects in the tray and observes the child's passage through distinctive phases of healing. While many child therapists use sand play in their therapy, this type of play therapy stands alone, embedded in its own theory and technique.

THE TECHNIQUES OF CHILD THERAPY

The theoretical frameworks highlighted earlier—the psychoanalytic, existential, behavioral, and Jungian—are the major frameworks for conducting child therapy; almost every known technique can be subsumed under one of these head-ings. It is important to distinguish between the child therapies and the child therapy techniques. The child therapies are based on a theoretical framework; the techniques are chosen to implement therapy based on those conceptual frameworks. Some of the child therapies are flexible enough to incorporate a variety of techniques whereas others restrict the therapeutic approach.

DIRECTIVE VERSUS NONDIRECTIVE PLAY THERAPY

Yet another way to categorize the types of therapy employed with children is to differentiate between directive and nondirective styles of play therapy. Nondirective or client-centered play therapy, promoted by the relationship therapists, is nonintrusive; it parallels the client-centered approach created by Carl Rogers (1951). Axline (1969) is credited with the creation of this specific kind of play therapy, and she distinguished between nondirective and directive therapy by simply stating, "Play therapy may be directive in form—that is, the therapist may assume responsibility for guidance and interpretation—or it may be nondirective; the therapist may leave responsibility and direction to the child" (p. 9). The child is allowed and encouraged to choose the toys to play with and is given the freedom to develop or terminate any particular theme. Guerney (1980) cites two major features of client-centered therapy: First, the client-centered approach is "viewed as promoting the process of growth and normalization" and, second, the therapist "must rely on the child to direct this process at his or her own rate" (p. 58). The non-directive therapist observes the child's play, often affirming verbally what is seen. Guerney states, "The realization of selfhood via one's own map is the goal of non-directive play therapy" (p. 21).

The nondirective therapist cultivates hypotheses that are tested over time; interpretations are used sparingly and then only after a great deal of observation. Nondirective therapists give the child concentrated attention and refrain from answering questions or giving directives. Axline (1964) demonstrates the use of nondirective therapy in her classic work *Dibbs in Search of Self.* Nondirective techniques are always helpful in the diagnostic phase of treatment and, as Guerney (1980) points out, have been shown to be effective with a wide range of problems.

The basic difference between the nondirective and directive approaches rests in the clinician's activity in the therapy. Directive therapists structure and create the play situation, attempting to elicit, stimulate, and intrude upon the child's unconscious, hidden processes or overt behavior by challenging the child's defensive mechanisms and encouraging or leading the child in directions that are seen as beneficial. Nondirective therapists are "actually controlled, always centered on the child, and attuned to his/her communications, even the subtle ones" (Guerney, 1980, p. 58). Directive therapies are by nature more short-term, more symptom-oriented, and less dependent on the therapeutic transference than are nondirective therapies.

The directive therapies are multitudinous and include, among other things, behavior therapies, Gestalt therapy, filial therapy, and family therapy. Certain specific techniques, such as puppet play, story-telling techniques, certain board games, and various forms of artistic endeavor, lend themselves to being employed in therapy in different ways: A nondirective therapist might provide the child with ample opportunities for art work or story telling with puppets whereas a directive therapist might ask the child to draw specific things or tell an exact story.

The Treatment of Abused Children

TREATMENT CONSIDERATIONS IN WORKING WITH ABUSED CHILDREN

When assessing the treatment needs of abused children and formulating treatment plans, it is vital to consider a number of issues such as, among other things, the phenomenological impact of the abuse, the family's level of dysfunction, the environmental stability, the age of the child, and the child's relationship to the offender.

The actual act of abuse is usually only one of myriad experiences the child endures. More often than not, the recognition and reporting of the abuse to the authorities sets into motion a number of legal and protective interventions that are perplexing and anxiety-provoking to the child. Consequently, the treatment of abused children is multidimensional and will likely include an array of services including individual, parent–child, group, and family therapy—all delivered within the context of social service and legal systems that operate within their own regulations and limitations.

The therapy of abused children includes the monitoring of risk factors, coordination with a variety of agencies, adherence to requests for periodic reports, and a focus on processing of the child and family's trauma, as well as intervention in intricate family dynamics, observation of parent–child interactions, work with foster families or other temporary caretakers for the child, advocacy efforts, testifying in court as needed, and other special activities that are discussed in the final chapter of this book.

The Phenomenological Experience

First and foremost, it is urgent to view each child's experience as unique. References were made to "mediators of abuse" earlier in this book, and there might be a temptation to judge the impact of abuse by certain yardsticks, such as the duration of the abuse, the severity, how many symptoms arise, who the perpetrator was, or how the child appears. The reality is that children react differently, and although the research can serve as a kind of global map of common repercussions, only close examination will reveal the subtle landmarks.

I once worked with a family of five children, ages two, four, seven, ten, and fifteen, whose home was burned down as a result of a freak gas explosion. The parents made swift and appropriate responses, buying the children duplicates of their favorite things, talking to them in a group about the experience, and bringing themselves and the children for some family counseling sessions. The parents commanded authority, coped well with their stress, and conveyed positive feelings to the children, centering on the fact that they had all survived and that that was the most miraculous and important thing. The parents also had the financial means to rent a comfortable home, and their insurance provided substantial compensation for erecting a new home. The children were involved in the plans and were awarded the right to "design" their own space if interested. The counseling sessions were almost redundant, since the parents had engaged the children in effective verbal communication. It was clear this was a close and communicative family, and their skills were well applied during the crisis. Some of the younger children's art work and play had elements of reenactment, as they drew fires and tumbled buildings. The children had also had fretful sleep, particularly the older ones, who seemed to have a greater understanding of how close they had come to death.

After six or eight conjoint meetings with the family, the parents and I agreed that I would be available to the children should any concerns arise in the future. Six months later the parents brought their 7-year-old son into therapy because he was unable to sleep, had lost his appetite (and 12 pounds), and appeared to go into alternating states of panic and what the parents described as "spacey" behavior—he sucked his thumb in the corner and had a fixed stare. In addition, he was afraid of the stove, the fireplace (which had not been used), and even the hot water in the tub. He flinched at any slight noise, and he had stopped playing outside. His brothers and sisters were not able to elicit his participation in either conversation or play. This is an example of how the same event, with subsequent similar responses, can be experienced differently by one child than by others when there has been no previous indication of marked personality differences among the children. The only explanation is the phenomenological nature of an individual's perception, integration, and processing of single or cumulative events, and this uniqueness commands great respect.

No matter what initial intervention is made, there is an inherent advantage in setting the therapeutic context for future work. Many of my child clients have had "discontinuous therapy," which allows and encourages families to return to therapy for "checkups" on an as-needed basis. However, it is my belief that the sooner a trauma victim enters treatment, the better.

Terr (1990) is quick to point out how quickly children and their families can recover from a trauma and cautions against postponing treatment:

> Putting off treatment for trauma is about the worst thing one can do. Trauma does not ordinarily get "better" by itself.

It burrows down further and further under the child's defenses and coping strategies. Suppression, displacement, overgeneralization, identification with the aggressor, splitting, passive-into-active, undoing, and self-anesthesia take over. The trauma may actually come to "look" better after all these coping and defense mechanisms go into operation. But the trauma will continue to affect the child's character, dreams, feelings about sex, trust, and attitudes about the future. (p. 293)

All presuppositions about abused children must be halted in the face of a new child victim. Assuming a child feels angry, sad, betrayed, depressed, or anything else is counterproductive. We must enter the assessment phase free from biases about the *general* effects of victimization or traumatization and enter the realm of learning from each child's singular experience. Only the children can tell or show us what meaning the experience has had to them. Only they can allow us to understand the incredible survival instincts of victims/survivors. They will show or tell us what they need although verbal directives are few and far between.

The clinician must set aside his/her own agenda and treatment plans must be individually designed and revised on a continuous basis.

The Family's Level of Dysfunction

The therapist may or may not have access to the abusive family when work is done with abused children. Abusive families, particularly neglectful ones, are frequently multi-problem families with high levels of dysfunction.

Even if the clinician has access to the family, their level of functioning might be so low as to minimize the impact of therapy. Therefore, it becomes critical for the clinician to lower expectations and devise realistic goals. Also, the clinician must take great care to ascertain how the child's progress is viewed at home. For example, the clinician may encourage the child to express his/her feelings and send the child into an environment where verbalizing feelings will elicit punishment. If the family is unresponsive and continues to organize around multiple crises, the most helpful interventions will be those designed to help the child cope with the realities of the environment.

Monitoring Risk Factors

Providing therapy to abused children, particularly those who have not been removed from their families, involves a special focus on risk factors to both the parents and the child clients. As Green (1988) notes, "Any plan for the treatment of child abuse must be designed to create a safe environment for the child and to modify the potentiating factors underlying the maltreatment...An effective treatment program must deal specifically with the parental abuse-proneness, the characteristics of the child that make him vulnerable, and the environmental stress that triggers the abusive interaction" (p. 859). It is therefore obligatory to have a clear understanding of the factors that led to the abuse and to have done a comprehensive review of these factors with the parents. For example, if one of the precipitators of the abuse was a parent's alcohol abuse, efforts must be made to monitor the parent's adherence to alcohol treatment programs. If one of the conditions of the court is that the child attend a daily child care program, it is important to verify that this is, in fact, transpiring. If the parental treatment is being conducted by another clinician, the child's clinician is advised to obtain contact with the relevant professionals and coordinate the risk management aspect of the therapeutic intervention.

Environmental Stability

As mentioned earlier, abusive families characteristically have a wide range of problems. They may have housing problems or frequent relocations, live in shelters, or even be homeless. The primary focus of the treatment is on providing the family and the child with as much information on resources and coping skills as possible. Clinicians who choose to work with abusive families must familiarize themselves with the multitude of prevention and treatment programs that have surfaced over the past 15 years. Up-to-date information is provided by local Child Abuse Councils, easily found in the

telephone directory. In addition, a National Child Abuse
Hotline maintains current resource information (1-800-4-A-
CHILD).

The Age of the Child

It is difficult to conduct play therapy with children under the
age of two. Two- to three-year-olds differ immensely in cognitive, motor, and verbal abilities. Children in this age group
should be assessed to determine how amenable they are to
therapy. Little is written about the treatment of young
children, although a number of professionals are beginning
to gain and share their expertise (MacFarlane, Waterman, et
al., 1986). Even children this young can exhibit posttraumatic play and reveal unconscious fears and concerns
through their play.

The Child's Relationship to the Offender

As noted earlier, the closer the relationship between the child
and the offender, the more potentially traumatic the event is
to the child. The clinician is once again advised to tread
lightly, suspending personal judgments about the child's
perpetrator. The child must sense that any and all feelings
he/she may have about the perpetrator are acceptable to the
clinician.

If, however, the child appears to be fixated on just one
feeling, the clinician can comment on that and gently direct
the child to other possible emotions. I once saw a young girl
who had been virtually abandoned by her mother and had
only sporadic contact with her. She was adamant that she
hated her mother, thought she was useless, and never
wanted to have anything to do with her. One day I softly said,
"You are really good at telling me about how angry you are
at your mother. And I bet you would be just as good at telling
me some of the other feelings you have or have had towards
her." She quickly retorted, "I don't feel anything else about
her." I added, "Maybe not now, but I bet when you were little
there might have been some other feelings." "Well yeah,

'cause I didn't know any better." Then I proceeded to ask what those feelings had been, and she cried a little as she described memories of wanting to go everywhere with her mother, and of feeling worried about her when she went out drinking. Just because a child emphasizes one primary feeling doesn't mean that other feelings might not be just beneath the surface.

Another child, also overtly hostile toward his mother, was unresponsive to queries about other feelings. I brought out my cards with "feeling pictures" (Communication Skillbuilders, 1988) and fanned them out in my hands. "Pick one," I prompted. When he did I asked him to tell me a time he had felt the (chosen) feeling about his mom. Because it was a game and there were explicit rules, the child simply acquiesced, and a lot of rich material sprang forward.

Treatment of the Child in His/Her Environment

Another difference in treating this population is the frequent instability of the environment. Often children are placed in foster homes (or a series of foster homes), group homes, or residential facilities. I have had more than one treatment interrupted by an abrupt transfer of my child client to another county or state.

Foster homes differ in quality. I have had contact with many highly qualified professionals, who have become part of the treatment team. Children who are removed from their home suffer the additional impact of separation from parents and familiar environments and usually need help dealing with separation anxiety, concern for their parents, and loyalty conflicts (Itzkowitz, 1989).

The therapy must include an assessment of the child's environment and an attempt to coordinate informational exchange with the alternative family on a regular basis. My experience has been that most foster parents welcome contact with the therapist, appreciate being regarded as a member of a professional team, offer many valuable insights, and respond well to suggestions regarding the child. Too often, foster families or other caretakers are not contacted, and helpful information is unavailable to the clinician.

Discontinuous Therapy

As mentioned previously, working with abused children may include intermittent participation from the child. Parents may withdraw the child from treatment once the court mandate is no longer present, or financial restrictions may influence the parent's decision to terminate the therapy. In addition, the child may use the therapy well for a period of time and later shift to periods when she/he does not seem to want to come or does not engage in therapeutic play. These are but some of the circumstances that can precipitate the use of discontinuous therapy. Nevertheless, children can benefit greatly from these short-term, task-focused, involvements with therapy.

The Clinician's Gender

Children who are abused may develop idiosyncratic responses to persons of the same sex as their abusers, including clinicians. In some instances it may be advantageous to transfer the child so this issue can be resolved. For example, I worked with a boy victim who was raped by his father for over a year. This child was in therapy with me for over 2 years, became well adjusted to his long-term foster placement, processed the trauma issues, and developed a sense of competence, safety, and well-being. The combination of a safe environment and therapy worked wonders; yet the boy always shied away from men and, I observed, exhibited startle responses when he saw a male therapist in my office. His play indicated a reticence toward men and a preference for contact with women. Unfortunately, the foster parent was an unmarried woman and the boy's teachers had been women, except for the physical education teacher. The boy wanted to avoid physical education because of the teacher, and the school gave him a special dispensation based on his history. Thus, the child had effectively managed to expel all men from his life.

I decided to transfer the boy to a male therapist. At first he resisted vehemently, but the joint sessions with the male therapist intrigued him, and slowly but surely, I could see him explore the boundaries of the new situation, asking questions of the male therapist, handing him toys, and making definitive statements about his preferences. Finally, the day came for his first "alone" visit with the male therapist; I waited outside the office at a designated place. He came out of the office twice to make sure I was there but tolerated the visit fairly well. The therapy continued for another year, and even though I felt the child had already made great strides, his progress with the male therapist was very rewarding. The child became physically active, appeared to grow due to his more erect stature, and joined a soccer team. He no longer avoided men and had established a good relationship with the soccer coach.

Symptoms of Distress and Treatment Modalities

Relatively little has been written about the treatment of young abused children although the past 2 years has seen a welcome surge in books about therapy with sexually abused and traumatized children (Friedrich, 1990; James, 1989; Johnson, 1989; Terr, 1990). Treatment of sexually abused children has probably been the most widely researched and documented aspect of treatment of abused children, and many of these findings are applicable to victims of other types of abuse. Long (1986), for example, discusses relevant issues in the treatment of sexually abused children: importance of teaming with the child's mother; inappropriate attachment behavior; infant regressive behavior; need for body contact and body awareness; and need for education on feelings. All of these areas are addressed in treatment of abused and neglected children in general. Porter, Blick, and Sgroi (1982), referring to the psychological issues that must be dealt with in work with sexually abused children, list "damaged goods" syndrome, guilt, fear, depression, low self-esteem, poor social skills, repressed anger, and hostility. Added to these are traits most characteristic of incest victims: impaired ability to trust, blurred role boundary and role confusion, and pseudomaturity coupled with failure to accomplish developmental tasks, self-mastery, and control. Again, all victims of child abuse and neglect will benefit from the clinician's focus on these matters. Burgess, Holstrom, and Mc-Causland (1978) emphasize the importance of decreasing the child's anxiety and attempting to engender trust as a first step in the treatment process. MacVicar (1979) stresses that sexually abused children often confuse sex with affection and need some help understanding sexuality. Waterman (1986), reviewing the literature on the treatment of sexually abused children, notes that many treatment modalities have been used, including family systems; a combination of behavior therapy for perpetrator, marital therapy, and family therapy; individual short- or long-term child therapy; group therapy; and art or play therapy. Terr (1990) notes that traumatized children are characterized by emotions of terror, rage, denial and numbing, unresolved grief, shame, and guilt. She also states that such children develop "traumatophobia," or fear of fear itself. This fear that springs from psychic trauma, she says, "makes arch conservatives out of formerly flexible children" (p. 37). Beezeley, Martin, and Alexander (1976), in a study of 12 physically abused children who stayed in treatment over one year, found that children's improvement was seen in increased ability to trust, increased ability to delay gratification, increased self-esteem, increased ability to verbalize feelings, and increased capacity for pleasure. Beezley and associates found that progress was greatest if the parents were willing to let the child make changes and were willing to make changes themselves and if the therapist could influence the environment, that is, the school setting, the playroom, and the child's relationships with others (p. 210). Mann and McDermott (1983) point out that the common areas of psychological disturbance requiring clinical attention are fear of physical assault or fear of abandonment, leading to depression and anxiety; failure to meet parents' distorted expectations, leading to defective object relationships, struggles over dependency, and internalization of a "bad child" self-image with poor self-esteem; difficulty achieving separation and autonomy; and prolonged and heightened separation anxiety and ambivalence over attachment to caretakers as a result of multiple rejections and out-of-home placements, including hospitalizations (p. 285).

I can't imagine a situation in which an abused child would not require or benefit from individual therapy. The experience of victimization or traumatization is painful, alarming, and confusing enough to warrant speedy intervention. The individual therapy, which includes an ongoing assessment, may be short-term and may precipitate the need for family or group work. However, in my view, every abused child deserves a one-on-one experience with a trained professional.

At the same time, if the child is to be reunited with a formerly abusive family—whether it be physical or sexual abuse, neglect, or emotional maltreatment—it becomes requisite to see the family with the child present. In addition, if the child has been abused outside the home, the entire family experiences the impact of the traumatic event, and all members require assistance.

Probably nowhere else is the direct observation of the parent–child relationship as indispensable as it is in situations of child abuse. Many inexperienced clinicians have been baffled to learn of a new abusive incident after the parents had religiously reported that they were using better disciplinary techniques and had not engaged in overt conflicts. A parent can state that she/he has been making calm and reasonable requests of a child, but direct observation may lead to a different conclusion. The clinician may find that while some improvement has been made, the tone and pitch of the parent's voice, combined with nonverbal communication, continue to be harsh enough to terrify the child and discourage voluntary compliance.

Family therapists encourage the presence of all family members in therapy sessions, but they have been considerably lax in demonstrating methods for conducting family sessions with very young children (Scharff & Scharff, 1987). The most typical family therapy scenario consists of the family therapist meeting with the adults in the family while the young children are relegated to the corner with toys or drawing materials. Scharff and Scharff (1987) discuss family therapy with very young children, offering interesting and useful suggestions (p. 285).

Social Service Agencies and the Courts

Working with abusive families often necessitates contact with court and social service agency personnel, who are responsible for overseeing the protection of the child. This type of contact can be seen as an act of treason by parents who are nonvoluntary therapy clients. In order to maximize the chances of forming a therapeutic alliance (often an oxymoron) with these clients, I usually limit my contact with social service agencies to written communications and show the letters to my clients prior to mailing. In this way, triangulation can be avoided and the clients may feel less helpless. It's probably too much to expect that this simple action will elicit total trust, but most clients respond well to this method of compliance with the authorities.

In working with abusive families and children, it is important to ascertain what the authorities expect from them. In other words, what specific behaviors or activities does the court or social service agency expect from the family to avoid the child's removal or to bring about reunification. Behavioral objectives, rather than broad goals, must be outlined. For example, "The parents should get along better" is vague and can be better explained with an explicit statement like "The parents must stop hitting and begin to have communication with each other, resulting in at least two decisions a week about the children and two decisions a week about how to spend their money." This specificity will greatly aid the clinician in assessing progress and in implementing treatment in a purposeful way.

Confidentiality and the Reporting Law

The mental health professional encounters a serious dilemma when treating allegedly abused or identified abused children. The dilemma originates because clinicians create an environment where, hopefully, a child feels safe and comfortable enough to share his/her inner thoughts, worries, or fears. When this atmosphere is accomplished by competent professionals and the child verbally or nonverbally shares or signals that he/she is being abused, the therapist is legally obligated to convey that information to the authorities. The child may feel betrayed by this apparent breach of trust and may withdraw into the uncomfortable or familiar position of having to decide what information can and cannot be divulged. And yet the reality is that the child abuse law was developed as a mechanism to obtain necessary protection for vulnerable children.

I find it necessary and desirable to tell the children from the outset that there are limits to confidentiality, that clinicians have certain legal obligations that supersede the obligations of confidentiality. This can be done in a matter-of-fact way in simple language, for example: "Everything we talk about in here is private. I won't repeat things that you tell me to anyone unless I get worried about a few things. I will have to tell someone if I think you are hurting yourself, hurting someone else, or if someone is hurting you, including your parents or brothers and sisters. 'Hurting' means different things like hitting or touching on private parts of the body." Then the child should be encouraged to ask questions or get further clarification. The clinician's answers should be confined to what is known. One of the ways that children will definitely feel betrayed is if the clinician predicts or promises a particular outcome, for example, the child will or will not stay at home or protective services or police will or will not come to the school.

Regardless of how many steps are taken to minimize the impact of a child abuse report, the child almost always regrets saying anything, particularly if the abuser is someone the child loves or depends on. The clinician must be sensitive to the child's predicament and avoid using false reassurances such as, "Everything will be all right now."

The Legal System

Probably one of the most disheartening aspects of therapy with abused children is the unpredictability and length of certain legal procedures. If the child must testify, this process can feel endless to the professionals—to say nothing of the children themselves. There are frequent continuances, and even when the child is required to testify, busy calendars or other external factors can require the child to return again and again before he/she is actually put on the stand.

Clinicians are sometimes criticized by defense attorneys for "preparing" a child to testify. A child's testimony can be discredited if she/he states that the testimony has been discussed with a therapist beforehand. Because of this, I suggest that the content of the child's testimony not be discussed during therapy sessions. The clinician can be helpful, however, in preparing the child to go to court. Caruso (1986) developed a set of pictures depicting a courtroom, the judge, the waiting room, and where the child sits. These pictures can familiarize the child with the courtroom ambience. In particular, the child should have some concrete idea of where she/he will sit to testify and of the distance from the offender; it is helpful if children who will testify know that they will be face-to-face with the offender, will likely be asked to identify the person, and can look at their own attorney or anywhere else if looking at the offender feels awkward or disturbing.

Court-Mandated Evaluations. A child's treatment is customarily suspended when the court requests an "independent" evaluation and is resumed once the evaluation is completed. The child's therapist and the evaluator prepare the child for the evaluation process, clearly explaining the projected length. Suspending the child's treatment sessions during the evaluation process may maximize the evaluator's potential to obtain important information from the child. There are circumstances in which suspending treatment might be contraindicated.

Report Writing. Working with abused children and their families can often be accompanied by nagging subpoenas for records. It has become my practice to write brief, matter-of-fact notes limited to issues of concern regarding the protection of the child. It is also my practice to always make every effort to protect my client's confidentiality, making phone calls to my attorney in attempts to "block" subpoenas while remaining fully cooperative.

Testifying. Yet another customary adjunct in the therapy of abused children is the possibility of the clinician's having to give depositions or testify in court. These are always distracting and stressful, no matter how well accustomed the clinician becomes to them. Recent information, indispensable to clinicians who serve as expert witnesses or provide other testimony in court, has become available (Myers et al., 1989). I advise the clinician to secure an attorney well versed in issues of family custody.

Advocacy Efforts. Finally, working with abused children may precipitate a number of concerns regarding the social service and legal system and how it operates. Some clinicians find it worthwhile to channel some of their concerns into letters to the legislature, participation in statewide organizations dedicated to these issues, or membership in local child abuse councils.

Working with abused children and their families is challenging, stressful, and quite an opportunity. There are a number of obstacles, and planning ahead will prevent many of the typical problems associated with this work such as not knowing what's expected, getting involved in interagency conflicts, learning suddenly that new workers have been assigned to the case, and feeling helpless and futile. The clinician will be most successful working as part of a team, talking with other professionals on a regular basis, asking for guidelines in writing, and meeting periodically to discuss the status of the case.

APPLICATION OF ESTABLISHED CHILD THERAPIES TO WORK WITH ABUSED CHILDREN

At no other time in history has the child therapy field had such a rich array of therapeutic tools and props for therapists to use. This is likely in response to the increase in childhood problems (such as drug abuse, delinquency, child abuse, suicide, youth prostitution) and a greater awareness within the mental health profession and the general public of the need for and efficacy of therapy for childhood problems. Clinicians currently working with abused children are in the enviable position of being able to draw from a growing literature reflecting many professionals' ground breaking and dedicated work. This cumulative knowledge helps us design more sensitive and effective treatment programs.

Some of the established child therapies are applicable to the therapy of abused children. These children have challenged mental health professionals with an array of unique behaviors that command a specialized response. The interventions are not offered as rigid, inflexible, or final in any way. The field of play therapy in general, and play therapy with abused children specifically, is in evolution; as more and more clinicians become trained and experienced and as research findings shape our understanding and thinking, more directives will be available about effective therapeutic strategies. The truth is that currently there are very few "rules" about this type of treatment, and we must equip ourselves with as much knowledge and experience as possible.

THE TREATMENT PLAN

As mentioned earlier, abused children are referred to treatment with an assortment of clinical symptoms that manifest underlying issues. The fundamental goal of therapy is to provide *corrective* and *reparative* experiences for the child. A corrective approach provides the child with the experience of safe and appropriate interactions that engender a sense of safety, trust, and well-being. In other words, there is an attempt to demonstrate to the child through therapeutic intervention the potentially rewarding nature of human interaction. A reparative approach is designed to allow the child to process the traumatic event in such a way that it can be consciously understood and tolerated. The healing power of play cannot be underestimated; likewise, the survival instinct of humans cannot be underrated. If given a nurturing, safe environment, the child will inevitably gravitate toward the reparative experience. Even in the unfortunate situation where children are kept in actively abusive homes, or returned prematurely after temporary foster care, the reparative clinical experience tends to be stored and remembered, later serving as a motivating factor. Of course, the impact of the reparative experience will depend on many external factors, such as the degree of continuity in the therapeutic setting, how well parents or caretakers cooperate, and how rigorous the efforts of social service agencies and courts are in planning for the child's future.

When a treatment plan is being designed for an abused child, the presenting symptoms must not be considered in isolation. Beginning efforts are appropriately directed toward the reduction of the child's symptoms, but therapeutic efforts must persist long after the relief of symptomatology. Too many children are terminated hastily by relieved parents or shortsighted clinicians.

As stated previously, each child is unique and treatment plans will vary according to the child's needs, level of damage, ongoing response to therapy, and accessibility. In the following pages I discuss various treatment areas and include specific therapeutic suggestions for each area.

Relationship Therapy

Because abuse is interactional and usually occurs within the framework of a family, the child can profit from an opportunity to experience a safe, appropriate, and rewarding interaction with a trusted other.

Children entering treatment are curious, reticent, and often anxious or afraid. Physically or sexually abused children, or children who have witnessed domestic violence, have a background that can predispose them to feeling vulnerable. They have learned that the world is unsafe and have met the challenge by cultivating such defensive mechanisms as hypervigilance or extreme compliance. The neglected child, conversely, may show little resistance to coming to therapy and may appear uninterested in and unaffected by the new surroundings. The neglected child is accustomed to inattention and has probably lacked even the most basic stimulation; he/she may sit still, expecting little. It is important in these cases for the clinician to underwhelm the child, then gradually introduce more stimulation. For example, sitting next to the child, facing away, coloring, or playing with some objects may be a good beginning; then, commenting on what is being done, directing the child's attention to toys, and, eventually, facing the child, asking questions, and encouraging the child's participation in a simple task like coloring will be effective.

The clinician always proceeds with caution, gingerly laying a foundation that advances a sense of security. (I have often imagined this step as the creating of a kind of sanctuary: quiet, accepting, stable, consistent, and free of external conflict.) One of the ways to create a sense of safety is to have a stable structure so the child can rely on certain aspects being constant.

Structure means many things. The length of the session, the location, the toys in the playroom, the "rules," the therapist's presence, and the procedure followed during the therapy hour are all features that can be used to build a strong structure. Even the way the therapist introduces himself/herself to the child is carefully designed. I have always found it best to be short and to the point in all communications with children:

My name is Eliana. I am someone who talks and plays with children. Sometimes I talk to kids about their thoughts and feelings. Other times, I play whatever the child wants.

Regarding rules I say the following:

There are lots of things you can do in here. You can play with anything you see. You can talk if you want. You can play or draw. You choose what to do. Sometimes I might ask you some questions. You can answer or not.

There are a few rules. No hitting or breaking toys. No hurting yourself or me. All the toys stay here.

We'll meet together for 50 minutes. I'll set this timer and when the bell goes off, it's time to stop until next time.

Everything we talk about is private. I won't tell anybody what you say unless you are hurting yourself, hurting someone else, or someone is hurting you, including your parents or brothers or sisters. If that happens, I'll need to tell someone else so we can make sure you're OK, but I'll talk to you about it first.

Obviously, all these rules are not announced in the first session. In that session I usually introduce myself and give the general directives for what will happen. After that, I scatter the rules throughout the succeeding sessions.

The clinician focuses on the child's needs and provides the child with opportunities for self-exploration, adaptation, and new (functional) behaviors. The nondirective, client-centered therapies are most beneficial at the beginning of treatment. The child is respected and accepted. The child chooses what to do and what to talk about. The therapist observes (actively) and documents the child's behavior, affect, play themes, interactions, and so on. The therapist makes a great effort to earn the child's trust, responds honestly, does what is promised, and is present week after week.

The therapist must resist the temptation to overgratify or overstimulate the child; compliments and overattention must be curtailed. Factual statements are best. "You have new shoes on today" might be a more productive statement than "Your new shoes are beautiful." It's always better to inquire how children view something, as opposed to telling them how they feel. "How do you like your new shoes?" is more conducive to communication than "I bet you love your new shoes." These children may find it difficult to disagree with an adult's opinion.

Likewise, if questions are necessary (and sometimes they are), they must be phrased to avoid a yes/no response.

It can be difficult to make the transition to open-ended questions, but the results are most helpful to children. In addition, I have learned through trial and error the relative merits of using comments rather than questions—comments that invoke the child's interest. My favorite and most successful comment is "Humm, I wonder what that might be like...." or "I wonder what other feelings might be there...." Given the implied freedom to wonder along, children may freely offer their own thoughts.

Assuming the therapeutic structure is well received and the child begins to attend sessions more voluntarily—perhaps even looking forward to them—the child may discern positive regard from the clinician. Now the challenge commences, since abused children have frequently learned that intimacy implies threat.

One of the insidious lessons of physical, sexual, or emotional abuse is that "people who love you will hurt you." Neglected children learn that "people who love you abandon you." Either way, intimacy implies threat, and the child who feels reassured or consoled will inevitably feel endangered. Feeling in peril, the abused child may attempt to take flight emotionally, physically, or through some acting-out behavior. Understanding the child's need to flee or need to evoke an abusive response from the clinician provides direction for the clinician's serene and persistent responses. Green (1983) has postulated that the tendency of the child to provoke abuse may serve a need to "obtain otherwise unavailable physical contact and attention" (p. 92).

One memorable 6-year-old brought me a paddle four months into treatment. "What's this?" I asked. "It's a paddle," she said, surprised by the question. "What's it for?" I continued. "For you to hit me," she announced. I looked puzzled, stating, "Why would I want to hit you?" Her response was simple. "You like me, don't you?" It was as simple and as sad as that. She assumed that my regard for her would be followed by an attack. Rather than tolerate the anticipatory anxiety of waiting for the attack, she decided to take the initiative and provide me with my weapon. Needless to say, the next four months in therapy were quite a trial of wills.

She kept provoking and I continued to simply state, "I am not going to hit you, yell at you, or get mad. I'm going to show you that I care about you in different ways." I also said, "You would really feel much better if I hit you or screamed at you right now. But that is something that will not happen. I know that you expect grown-ups will hurt you, and I also know that you will learn that I will not hit or hurt you." The little girl needed to learn to tolerate the anxiety of expecting an attack. When I noticed her tension, I would say, "You're feeling worried that I might hurt you right now...it's OK to worry a little, until you know deep down that you'll be safe." Other times I would say, "I know you're worried, and it's OK to tell me when you feel that way. Sometimes, after you worry for a little while and nothing happens to you, the worry gets smaller and smaller." At the end of therapy she made me a little stitched purse and gave me a card saying, "Eliana. Thanks for liking me and not hitting me. Your friend always."

For neglected or needy children, the wish for attachment may loom strongly. These children make indiscriminate connections and seem desperate to be special to the therapist. They may ask point-blank, "Do you like me the best of all the children you see?" or "Do you miss me when I'm not here?" For them, intimacy is not encumbered with threatening feelings; it is an elusive sensation they long for. I respond to these questions by asking what they imagine I might feel and then commenting on how important being liked or missed is to them. If children persist I will say, "I do like you," "You are special," or "I think of you sometimes during the week" and then inquire what it's like for them to hear these things.

Setting limits for these children, by gently asserting the nature of the therapeutic relationship, is important. Not setting limits can be counterproductive for the child and his/her family. If the clinician becomes overly responsive to the child's needs or begins to behave in unusual ways (such as buying clothes and other presents for the child), the abusive or neglectful parent will be affected inadvertently. One therapist consulted with me when her 7-year-old client proclaimed, "I want you to be my mommy. I don't like my mommy as well as you." It is possible that a child could develop this feeling without *any* encouragement, and yet I have frequently met well-meaning therapists who regret that they failed to keep clear boundaries in the therapeutic relationship with the child (and who confide that keeping clear boundaries is more difficult with children).

The psychodynamic concept of "transference" has applicability in work with abused children. Scharff and Scharff (1987) reviewing Freud's concept of transference, explain that Freud defined transference as "the repetition of a psychological experience from the past applied to the person of the physician: The physician is simply the present site for the distribution of the libido, or sexual energy, of the patient" (p. 203). Transference, therefore, refers to the relocation of thoughts and feelings about a primary person in the child's life to the clinician. The abused child is liable to experience emotions such as distrust, fear, rage, and longing toward the clinician. These feelings originate in the parental relationship and get transferred to a person who may feel safer to the child or who may require less caretaking or loyalty. As a result the therapist must refrain from behaving in any set way. Some therapists who work with abused children allow countertransference issues to dictate their behavior.

As alluded to earlier, abused children may become anxious and threatened by the unfamiliar (nonabusive) behavior of the clinician. These children feel helpless or bewildered by nonabusive behaviors, and in an effort to feel more in control and less anxious, they may become provocative.

During my first internship with abused children I, in my inexperience, brought with me, out of countertransference needs, an enormous desire to be nurturing. Many of the children literally attacked me, kicking my shins, punching my arms, and biting me. Green (1983) has suggested that the compulsion to repeat trauma and the identification with the aggressor "replace[s] fear and helplessness with feelings of omnipotence" (p. 9). This attacking behavior from children can evoke disturbing responses in the clinician. It was when I first confronted this behavior that I first acknowledged, as I have often shared in lectures, having hostile feelings toward children. I later came to recognize these angry feelings not as a sign that I needed to find a new career but as a sign that the children were provoking responses in me that were familiar to them in an effort to take care of their needs. Probably the greatest lesson I have learned from abused children and adults is that everything they do after they have been abused is designed to keep themselves feeling safe. This concept is beneficial in evaluating even the most difficult or irritating behavior. While early in the treatment I simply document the child's responses, and set limits when needed, once the therapeutic relationship is established, I make my observations explicit by describing to the child the connection between his/her behavior and underlying issues.

Nonintrusive Therapy

Because physical and sexual abuse are intrusive acts, the clinician's interventions should be nonintrusive, allowing the child ample physical and emotional space.

Physical and sexual abuse are intrusive acts that violate the child's boundaries. The body is hit or penetrated and the child feels "too much" of the parent. In these families abuse can be accompanied by emotional encroachment or detachment, either of which makes the abuse more complex. Abused children frequently have the experience of having extreme and unreasonable directives about what to think, what to feel, and what to do. The parents are either enmeshed with or disengaged from the child and may either restrict the child from any privacy or be totally apathetic. An abusive parent may sporadically want to take care of all the child's hygiene needs whereas a neglectful parent may fail to oversee any of the child's hygiene practices. Moreover, the behaviors of abusive and neglectful parents can fluctuate, particularly when drug or alcohol abuse is involved.

Because of these boundary problems the clinician's early interventions should be nonintrusive, allowing the child to set the boundaries. The child should be allowed to move around freely and choose desired activities. While the child plays, the therapist is advised to sit nearby, without hovering over the child's every movement. It is best to avoid a question and answer format and, instead, allow the child to communicate spontaneously as desired. The clinician may obtain valuable information immediately. For example, some children may throw things, break things, wander in and out of the room, reset the timer, and generally test all of the regulations defiantly. Other children do the opposite: They sit quietly in a corner, avoiding interactions of any kind. They seem to recoil from the therapist, creating their needed seclusion; they are unresponsive and subdued. Sometimes these initial behaviors taper off after a while; at other times they linger beyond the expected period. All the child's behaviors are informative and purposeful. Both what the child does and what he/she fails to do furnish details of the child's inner world. If the child persists in a nonverbal mode or appears to feel pressured to perform verbally, the clinician may speak aloud, without addressing the child specifically. This technique is called "talking to the wall," and may allow a resistant child to listen in, and possibly respond. As the therapy proceeds it may be necessary to become more directive, particularly if the child continues to be avoidant or too guarded—especially about the abuse.

Some clinicians question what to do if the child avoids the topic of abuse in therapy. Often when I inquire into the details of the case, I find that the clinicians are relying on verbal validation of some kind. One clinician, who described the child's elaborate posttraumatic play, was frustrated that the child never made verbal reference to his abuse.

One of the errors in child therapy is observing the child passively rather than in an active mode. Active observation requires the therapist to participate in the child's play, not necessarily in a physical way but certainly in an emotional way. The therapist remains interested and involved, mentally logging the sequence of play, the themes, the conflicts and resolution, the child's affect, and the verbal commentary as it evolves.

The clinician must also refrain from inadvertently encouraging or permitting too much "random play," or play that has symbolic obstruction. A recent (and I hope short-lived) trend among therapists is to equip their offices with computer games: Children become absorbed in these games, but they are devoid of therapeutic usefulness. Therapists seem to use these games the same way parents do: to entertain and/or relax the child. Less obvious, but equally worthless, is outfitting the therapy room with popular toys, such as converters and electric cars. These toys will summon specific types of play in children and do not lend themselves to symbolic reenactment of internal concerns.

If the child is making good use of therapy, his/her play will be sporadically significant to the clinician; it will almost always be enriching for the child.

Ongoing Assessment

Probably in no other kind of therapy is an ongoing assessment so necessary. Children may unfold during therapy, sharing their emotions and feelings as they begin to trust. They are also in a state of continuous developmental change with accompanying personality transfigurations.

Unlike that of an adult client, a child's personality is maturing during the course of treatment. A child is often "in the midst of rapid and continuous developmental and environmental changes" (Diamond, 1988, p. 43). As Chethik (1989) elucidates, "The child's personality is in a state of evolution and flux," with an immature ego, fragile defenses, easily stimulated anxiety, and often feelings of magic and omnipotence (p. 5). The child's ego is expanding; his/her consciousness and self-consciousness are developing; he/she is tentatively establishing identities; and he/she develops a repertoire of defenses and coping skills. Depending on the length of treatment, children's transformation can be immense as they tackle the pertinent developmental tasks. Children are influenced greatly by peers, and their behavior may change drastically under the influence of friends or teachers. As a result therapy strategies must sometimes change to address these differences: A child who is suddenly defiant and challenging may require firm limits; a child who begins to question his/her competence may require a focus on simple tasks that result in success; a child who suddenly becomes extroverted and inquisitive may benefit from a therapist who responds in an informative and directive manner.

However, any and all changes in the clinician's strategies must be well thought out and *purposeful*. I have frequently told students of child therapy that a clinician should be able to explain why she/he did what was done or said what was said—and why it was done or said at a particular moment. This can be more difficult with children who are less inhibited about their thoughts, actions, and behaviors and can act more impulsively. The clinician has less response time, which requires the ability to say, "I don't know," "Let me think about that a minute," or "I think I have two thoughts about that; let me take a second."

Effective assessments also require clear and measurable treatment plans based on active observations. Making a treatment plan with clear, concrete *behavioral objectives* allows the clinician a way to gauge progress. As I intimated earlier, one of the most common errors in working with children is an unfortunate tendency to ignore the child's play. Some clinicians seem lulled into passive participation in the therapy hour with children, perhaps because play can be self-absorbing for the child; many children require sparse interactions during their play. Greenspan (1981) maintains that active observation occurs on a variety of levels, involving the physical integrity of the child; the child's emotional tone; how the child relates to the clinician; the child's specific affects and anxieties; the way the child uses the environment; thematic development of the child's play (the way themes are developed in terms of depth, richness, organization, and sequence); and the therapist's subjective feelings about the child (p. 15). As Cooper and Wanerman (1977) suggest, "allow yourself a growing fascination with and respect for the minutiae of human behavior" (p. 107). The clinician who documents these levels of information is by necessity involved in the therapy as an observer–participant. Unless the therapist assumes this role, he/she is disengaged and is not conducting therapy to its fullest potential. If the therapist finds that the child is no longer using the play in a therapeutic way, or is engaged in stagnated or random and disorganized play, the therapist must intervene. However, if the therapist begins to think that the child's behavior is crystal-clear, the therapy warrants review. Cooper and Wanerman (1977) caution: "Slow down when you feel that you are beginning to understand the meaning of a child's play behavior" (p. 107).

Facilitative Efforts

Because abused, neglected, or emotionally abused children are frequently under- or overstimulated, they lack the ability to explore, experiment, and even play. The clinician must facilitate these natural, now constricted or disorganized tendencies.

Children who have been physically or sexually abused may be anxious, hypervigilant, dissociative, depressed, and/or developmentally delayed. They may be socially immature and may rely on the environment for performance cues. They may have had emotionally barren environments or emotionally chaotic and inconsistent ones. In either case their natural tendencies toward play may be interrupted, leading to anxious, disorganized, or chaotic play.

The clinician is advised to inquire about the child's common play patterns before meeting with the child. Parents, foster parents, day-care providers, or teachers may be able to provide information about attention span, play preferences, and other relevant issues. This knowledge is then used in selecting the type of playroom or play materials to be made available to the child. The chaotic, disorganized child will need a more restrictive setting with fewer options. The restriction can be accomplished by providing a large open space with previously selected toys or a smaller room with a limited number of toys to choose from. The worst possible combination for a child with disorganized, frenzied play is a large room with numerous toys and activities for selection.

The understimulated child will probably do the same in either setting. With this child, the clinician is, by necessity, more directive, selecting the toys and encouraging the child's interest and play. The therapist first attempts to encourage the child by modeling play behaviors, thus giving tacit permission for the child's participation. If the child continues to retreat from the play, the therapist can slowly encourage the child more directly. One of the major functions of play "is to alter the raw, overwhelming affects that arise in children at times of anxiety and provide a natural vehicle for the expression of these affects" (Chethik, 1989, p. 14). A child's continued lack of involvement with play could signal a different kind of problem, and medical and neurological exams are indicated.

The selection of toys for play therapy is critical. Axline (1969) suggests a list of required materials, including the following:

> nursing bottles, a doll family, a doll house with furniture, toy soldiers and army equipment, toy animals, playhouse materials, including table, chairs, cot, doll, bed, stove, tin dishes, pans, spoons, doll clothes, clothesline, clothespins, and clothes basket, a didee doll, a large rag doll, puppets, a puppet screen, crayons, clay, finger paints, sand, water, toy guns, peg-pounding sets, wooden mallet, paper dolls, little cars, airplanes, a table, an easel, an enamel-top table for finger painting and clay work, toy telephone, shelves, basin, small broom, mop, rags, drawing paper, finger-painting paper, old newspapers, inexpensive cutting paper, pictures of people, houses, animals, and other objects, and empty berry baskets to smash. (p. 54)

Clearly, not all these items will be equally effective.

The doll house, family dolls, nursing bottles, puppets, and art materials are the necessary minimum.

In working with abused children, I have found the following toys or techniques to be repeatedly successful in encouraging the child's verbal or play communication:

- Telephones
- Sunglasses
- Feeling cards (i.e., illustrations of faces expressing feelings)
- Therapeutic stories
- Mutual story-telling techniques
- Puppet play
- Sand play
- Nursing bottles and dishes and utensils
- Video therapy

Telephones connote intimate verbal communication to the child. I usually sit with my back to the child and mimic the confidential tone used in a phone call. The child usually turns away through example, and a more private conversation can ensue.

Sunglasses are magical: Children believe that they become invisible once they put sunglasses on. Wearing them gives children a comfortable anonymity that can disinhibit their communications, particularly when they have been feeling embarrassed or reticent.

Therapeutic stories have been frequently used in child therapy in a convincing way. Because children's imagination and ability to identify is so powerful, they can easily enter a story, making unconscious connections to heroes, conflicts, and resolutions. Stories have been used to teach children some basic concepts and to encourage their interest through a familiar medium.

A wonderful book that offers therapeutic stories specifically for abused children was made available recently (Davis, 1990). The author, trained in Ericksonian hypnosis, found that the use of metaphors in therapy could directly engage the child's unconscious mind and facilitate lasting changes. Her stories, specifically designed for an array of child-related problems, are insightful and very effective, particularly with latency-age children and preadolescent youngsters (and in some instances younger children as well).

Gardner's (1971) Mutual Story-Telling Technique can also have good results, but it necessitates the creation of a story by the child. Some abused children have restricted creativity and are anxious about their performance, so this technique may be more successful later in therapy.

Puppet play has several benefits. The child creates a story but does so anonymously, so to speak, using specific characters to portray hidden conflicts or concerns. I find it especially useful to have a sheet the child can sit behind, so that she/he can conduct the play while hidden.

Sand play can be very evocative. Children tend to like the sand (maybe because it's reminiscent of beaches) and enjoy the tactile experience of molding and shaping it or simply letting it rain through their fingers. My impression is that some children use sand play as a way to feel nurtured or soothed; they feel calmed by the play. Other children immediately produce intricate scenarios, abundant with symbolism. The play is in and of itself therapeutic and provides the child with ample opportunities for a reparative experience.

The use of videos in therapy is very worthwhile. Abused children may be reticent to disclose their worries, fears, or self-doubts. They often have impaired self-images and lack the insight or confidence to recognize or express themselves freely. Watching videos that discuss topics such as self-esteem, emotional abuse, secrets, drug abuse, or coping with feelings, can be extremely beneficial for children for two reasons. First, it gives them a little distance to consider personal issues they may otherwise avoid, and second, the issue is presented in the child's medium, story-telling, and has the potential to engage the child's interest. I believe the first step toward self-empathy is the ability to empathize with others; the child watching a character in a videotape has the option to identify with the character, empathizing with his/her plight. The information presented in the tape is then discussed between the clinician and the child. I have been most impressed with a series created by J. Gary Mitchell (MTI Productions, 1989) in which a character called "Super Puppy" guides children through a variety of important issues such as those mentioned previously.

It's worth noting that children with established play patterns find it essential to have toys available to them on a consistent basis. Toys must be protected and constancy maintained. Toys do not leave the playroom under any circumstances. In addition, the therapist must convey a sense of comfort with the child's use of the toys (I have met therapists who buy expensive or irreplaceable antiques for the playroom, creating a kind of museum.)

Expressive Efforts

Because abused children are frequently forced or threatened to keep the abuse secret, or somehow sense that the abuse cannot be disclosed, efforts must be made to invite and promote self-expression.

Sundry ways of stimulating expression must be undertaken. Art, sand play, storytelling, doll play are all useful attempts. However, a child who seems averse to overtly expressing himself/herself may require considerable effort.

One technique I've found fruitful is making the need and use of secrecy explicit. I mark a paper bag "Secrets" and play a game with the child in which, every now and then we each pull out one of the secrets written on folded pieces of paper. The child may choose to select another secret to read aloud. The child sees this as a game and has less resistance to disclosing scary or uncomfortable secrets.

Sometimes I draw cartoon figures, for example, of a small child and an adult placing an empty cloud above their heads the way cartoonists do. Then the child fills in what is being said.

Caruso's Projective Story-Telling Cards (1986) are also effective because they depict so many familiar situations for children who live in dysfunctional families. The characters are obviously experiencing conflict, danger, fear, or discomfort. Children have an opportunity to project their own worries or concerns into the characters in the drawing. The clinician learns about the child and responds to his/her concerns as the child's projected concerns become clear.

There are no strict rules about techniques that can be employed to encourage the child to reveal inner thoughts and feelings. The clinician must be as creative as possible, using whatever interest areas the child displays. Perhaps no other clinician contributed such a multitude of creative ideas as James (1989). The more numerous the techniques available, the better; abused children can be resistant to self-disclose for a variety of external and internal reasons.

My impression has been that many children have difficulty with the expression of anger. They are afraid of the emotion, probably because of their history. They need to see anger as a normal emotion that can be expressed constructively and safely, not just in inappropriate and dangerous ways.

Most abused children have resentments and feelings of anger; however, they frequently squelch these feelings to stay safe. Providing them with permission to show anger can generate a variety of experimental behaviors, some safer than others. It is useful to model safe expressions of anger, setting the necessary limits.

If the child shows more of a certain type of feeling than others, the clinician must begin to inquire about the range, for example, by saying, "You are very good at showing your angry feelings. What do you do when you feel sad?" Sometimes feelings are shown through the body. Children may tense up, bite their lip, or even scratch themselves during specific discussions in the therapy. The child's posture can help the clinician determine which concerns need attention.

Abuse affects the child physically. In physical abuse there is a great deal of pain sustained by the child; the body will develop physiologic responses, including muscle tension, and evidence of anxiety, such as flinching. An abused child, living with erratic violence, can literally prepare the body for an attack by holding the body still and experiencing other signs of physical distress such as shallow breathing, increased heart rate, and flushing. In cases of sexual abuse the child's body has usually been penetrated, creating a feeling of vulnerability. The child's body feels unsafe, and the sexually abused child does not have a sense of physical control.

Finally, some emotionally abused and neglected children do not receive normal physical attention or affection, and since it has been clearly demonstrated that physical nurturing of a child is as important as alimentation, neglected children can feel confused or inundated by a fear of or wish for touching.

Because of the innate physical issues for abused children, helping parents and caretakers encourage the child's physical activity is vital. The child needs to engage in the most basic of physical movements; walking, climbing, and running can begin to give the child a sense of accomplishment and pride as well as a knowledge of his/her physical limitations. It is important to keep expectations to a minimum until the child begins to thrive, allowing him/her to experiment at an individual pace.

When the child appears to be more physically comfortable, less tense, and more prone toward physical activity, it can be beneficial to enroll the child in some kind of team sport at school or through a park and recreation department. Participating in group activities can engender a sense of well-being and belonging.

In addition, the formerly abused child may find self-defense courses educational and worthwhile. The abused child who learns principles of self-defense may feel empowered and less threatened by the environment. Most of the self-defense classes do not teach violence; they teach self-protection and respect for others. There is a great deal of self-motivation and self-discipline involved in learning self-defense, and many children I've worked with have responded well to this instruction.

Although there are some sex differences regarding preference of activity (boys prefer self-defense, girls prefer dance or movement), children can be stimulated to develop other interests if the activity is normalized. For example, one boy who was in a group with two other boys who took dance classes, developed an interest in dance classes after meeting other boys who liked this activity.

Directive Efforts

Abused or traumatized children may also have a tendency to try to suppress frightening or painful memories or thoughts and in some cases may use denial and avoidance fully.

Suppression is a necessary defense that allows the individual to store intolerable material in the unconscious so that it no longer interferes with current functioning.

Eventually, the abused child will be served by being able to suppress or consciously inhibit a specific impulse, idea, or affect associated with the trauma, but traumatic memories are best suppressed after they have been processed and understood. When this is done the individual has fewer experiences with fragmentation or splitting and dissociation. It is the repressed, or unconsciously stored memories, that can leak out into consciousness through posttraumatic symptoms.

The child's first and most natural tendency will be to use the defense of denial or suppression; the family frequently joins in to try to put the unpleasant or painful memory behind. Families can reorganize quickly after a trauma, taking care to avoid individuals or situations that can trigger the memory.

The therapist can help a child who is avoiding the processing of traumatic material by guiding him/her through a thorough, time-limited review of the traumatic event so that the event can be understood, felt, processed, and assimilated. It appears that no matter how long this process is postponed, eventually (for most people) the unconscious brings the event back to consciousness through symptoms of posttraumatic stress syndrome, including flashbacks, nightmares, auditory hallucinations, or behavioral reenactment.

There is growing evidence in the literature that many adult survivors have amnesia for the abuse for most of their lives. This indicates how powerful and effective the defense mechanisms can be. I believe we can give abused and traumatized children a real advantage if we stimulate their processing of the trauma. This does not mean that these children won't need different levels of explanation and reassurance as they become more cognitively and emotionally mature. It does mean that the foundation is set for future exploration.

Privacy

Because in-home physical and sexual abuse and neglect are family matters and children may feel loyal and protective of their parents, it is important to expect the child's reticence and to structure opportunities for him/her to divulge information at his/her own pace.

Some abused children are threatened by their families or caretakers to keep all family interactions to themselves. They are told that they or loved ones will be harmed. Some of the children I've worked with have had demonstrations of what will happen to them if they tell others about secret family situations. One child witnessed the murder of his dog. The parent threw the dog against a wall, and brutally crushed its head with a brick. This was the incident that precipitated the mother's taking flight with the child. The child suffered greatly about this for a number of years; since the child's environment was so wanting, the child had formed a strong tie with his pet.

Even when children are spared overt threats, many of them sense the secrecy of family violence or sexual abuse. They may not feel able to talk about feelings associated with their abuse.

Privacy is very important for children; secrecy is not. Establishing privacy empowers; keeping secrets engenders feelings of helplessness. Children required to keep secrets (through internal or external pressures) feel burdened, and the secret takes on great importance for them, alienating them from others and limiting the number of comfortable interactions they can have.

A number of techniques to clarify the difference between privacy and secrecy can be employed. Sometimes an abused child is at the crossroads of making a disclosure about disturbing thoughts or feelings. I might ask the child who refuses to continue, "What will happen if you say more?" If the child says "I don't know," I will explore possible alternatives by having the child "guess" what might happen. More frequently, the child has a specific reason for not telling, and she/he might respond, "Daddy will be mad at me" or "Mommy told me if I told, bad things would happen." I usually make the following statement, "It's really hard to talk about things when we're afraid. What might make it feel safer to talk about how you feel?"

Some children prefer to tell a stuffed animal in the playroom. I may ask them to pick out the animal they'd like to tell, and they can whisper it to them. Once they've done that, I ask how it feels to get these feelings out. Most of the time the children feel good about talking; sometimes they seem indifferent. I also might ask the child to imagine what the stuffed animal might say to them about their secret.

I have on occasion brought out a tape recorder and left the child alone in the playroom to tape what she/he wants to say but can't. Children usually ask if I will listen to the tape, and I answer that the tape belongs to them and they can let me listen when they want. Every time I've done this, the child has wanted to play the tape back to me right away. I then have an opportunity to comment about the secret. I might say something like "It must be hard to be alone with that secret" or "It must be hard to keep that just to yourself." I usually ask the child whom he/she might feel safer telling and continue to talk about the difficulties of keeping things to oneself.

Obviously, if the child's secret concerns an event such as physical abuse or sexual abuse, the reporting law may enter the picture. However, many of the secrets include situations that are burdensome to the child but not necessarily dangerous.

Posttraumatic Play

Because posttraumatic play often occurs in secret, the therapeutic environment must create a climate for this type of play. Once the play begins, it must be carefully monitored for alterations, and at some point interrupted with suitable interventions.

The traumatized child is often compelled to reenact the traumatic event in an effort to master it. This concept was first introduced by S. Freud as "repetition compulsion." As Terr (1990) has affirmed, the reenactments can take the form of behavioral manifestations as well as play dramatizations. A reenactment is usually the result of an unconscious compulsion that the child may not understand. Some children claim that no matter how much they try, they cannot stop thinking about the trauma and frequently feel as if it were "happening again." Others claim that they no longer remember anything about the traumatic event and stubbornly deny any and all feelings related to the event. Processing the trauma can be achieved in a variety of ways. Some children are more able to discuss their feelings and concerns and may ask disarming questions about their abuse.

Because play provides a medium for communication, some therapeutic play provides a mechanism for uncovering concerns and releasing pent-up feelings. Some children simply go about the task of doing what they need to do to feel better; they need little more than permission—and the props—to do so. When this happens the clinician can observe, document, and eventually comment on what transpires and answer the child's questions or concerns.

For other children—perhaps those who have been more harmed by the traumatic event—the clinician's direction and stimulation will be needed before the frightening or overwhelming feelings and sensations can be faced. In these cases, forming a solid therapeutic relationship precedes any gentle probing to assist the child in addressing intolerable emotions. The goal of this work is to allow the child eventually to process the traumatic event, give it appropriate and realistic meaning, and store it as a tolerable memory. It is unnecessary to force the child into endless work on the traumatic event, particularly when the child is not denying or avoiding but has now redirected psychic energy into developmental tasks.

The play of the traumatized child who reenacts is quite unique. The child ritualistically sets up the same panorama and acts out a series of sequential movements that result in the identical outcome. The posttraumatic play is very literal and devoid of apparent enjoyment or freedom of expression. The potential benefit of this play is that while the child is undergoing memories that are frightening or anxiety-provoking, she/he is going from a passive to an active stance, controlling the reenactment. In addition, the formerly overwhelming event is occurring while the child is in a controlled, safe environment. It is possible that the child gains a sense of mastery and empowerment from this type of play therapy. As Chethik (1989) says of a clinical example, "The repetitious play, the comments of the player–observer, and his own new solution helped him assimilate a past overpowering experience" (p. 61).

Posttraumatic play can remain fixed. Terr (1990) cautions that allowing a child to continue long-term posttraumatic play can be dangerous; the child may not release any anxiety, and may have feelings of terror and helplessness reinforced. For this reason, after observing that the posttraumatic play remains static for a period of time (eight to ten times), I attempt to intervene in the ritual play, in the following ways:

- Asking the child to make physical movement, such as standing up, moving arms, or taking deep breaths. Physical movement can free up emotional constriction.
- Making verbal statements about the child's posttraumatic play, suspending the self-absorption and rigidity of the play.
- Interrupting the sequence of play by asking the child to take a specific role, describing the perceptions and feelings of one of the players.
- Manipulating the dolls, moving them around, and asking the child to respond to "what would happen if..."
- Encouraging the child to differentiate between the traumatic event and current reality in terms of safety and what has been learned.
- Videotaping the posttraumatic play and watching the tape with the child, stopping it for discussion of what is observed.

The goal of interrupting posttraumatic play is to generate alternatives that might promote a sense of control, help the child express fragmented thoughts and feelings, and orient the child toward the future. It might take a number of interruptions before the child allows the intervention to change the posttraumatic play.

If the child is engaging in posttraumatic play at home and the parents or caretakers have noticed it, two possibilities exist: The clinician either makes a home visit and asks to witness the child's play directly or the clinician creates the posttraumatic scenario (as described by parents or caretakers) in the therapy hour. It is possible that the child dissociates during the posttraumatic play. Treatment strategies for dissociation (discussed later) must be implemented as well.

The child whose play is random, disorganized, and devoid of symbolism may need greater stimulation. If a child persists in failing to address the underlying issues naturally, the therapist, taking a directive position, must introduce the stimulus in the therapy. Several techniques can work. A puppet story told by the clinician in which the central character experiences the same trauma as the child may elicit a response. The child may empathize with the puppet's plight; empathy with others is a first step towards self-exploration and self-empathy.

Some attempts at desensitization may also work. One child I worked with was raped in a park, and yet she was unable to offer verbal or nonverbal communications regarding the trauma. Her silence was fueled by a fear that she had brought on the rape by going to the park when she should have gone directly home. The boys had told her she "wanted" to be raped, and she was very confused because she had indeed wanted to be noticed by the boys and had gone to the park to be seen by them after overhearing mention of their destination at school. I had the girl color a page in a coloring book that depicted a park; I created a park scene with dolls playing in a toy swing; I made a park in the sand. I drove by a number of parks and, finally, asked the girl to show me the park where she had been raped. We drove by it first, then sat in the car outside the park, then walked around the outside of the park, and finally walked inside. Once inside, when I stated that the boys were very wrong to rape her and hurt her, she cried almost instantly, saying repeatedly, "I was bad, I was bad." This session, and six or seven that followed, focused on the rape and the child's feelings of guilt and shame. Eventually, she understood that she had done nothing wrong and that wanting to be noticed by boys was perfectly natural. This child also benefited greatly by talking to another preteen who had also been a rape victim.

Allowing the child to simply reenact without any apparent resolution is, as Terr has noted, "dangerous." In addition, the repetition of a trauma without resolution will reinforce the child's sense of helplessness and lack of control. The clinician must take an active role in helping the child both enter and maneuver the play, a role of actively commenting, rearranging, or intruding upon the sequence of events the child portrays. Reexperiencing alone is not enough. The thoughts and feelings generated by the play must be acknowledged and discussed. In addition, the child needs a struc-

tured way of "debriefing" from the play once it has terminated. The clinician must take some time helping the child
reestablish a more comfortable emotional level. Guided im-
agery or simple relaxation techniques may have positive
results. Alerting the parents or caretakers to the difficult
work of the therapy, and asking them to plan appropriate
responses, is very important. During posttraumatic play the
child may appear more hypervigilant, anxious, and experience sleeping or eating disorders.

The overall goal of this work must be kept in the
forefront. As Scurfield (1985), describing his work with adult
survivors of various traumas, suggests the final step in the
stress recovery process is the integration of all aspects of the
trauma experience, both positive and negative, with the
survivor's notion of who he or she was before, during, and
after the trauma experience. Sours (1980), describing child
therapies, states that "child therapies in general, whether
they are supportive or expressive psychotherapies, tend to
rely on abreaction, clarification, manipulation, and the corrective emotional experience of the new object" (p. 273).

Treatment of Dissociation

*Victims of trauma may experience dissociation. The clinician
must assess for dissociation, and devise ways of addressing
the dissociative process.*

The DSM-III-R defines dissociation as "a disturbance or
alteration in the normally integrative functions of identity,
memory, or consciousness" (p. 269). Dissociation occurs along
a continuum; everyone experiences dissociative episodes,
such as highway hypnosis. Boredom, fatigue, or fear may
facilitate dissociation; the individual enters a trance state
that can last for brief or extensive periods of time. Sometimes
during frightening situations, like an earthquake, individuals may have brief dissociative episodes, later being
unable to remember specifically what happened, or how they
got from one place to another.

At the most extreme end of the dissociative continuum
is multiple personality disorder. Other less extensive forms

of dissociation include depersonalization, psychogenic amnesia, and fugue states. Depersonalization is very common among abuse victims. Children often describe "out of body" experiences, in which they feel as if they are floating on the ceiling. From that vantage point (while emotionally detached) they look down on themselves. The ability to dissociate allows the child to mentally escape the dangerous or threatening situation. At the same time, the child may become confused about his/her own identity, having trouble remembering what has occurred. Psychogenic amnesia, in fact, is a disturbance in memory. Many child and adult survivors are unable to remember specific events or periods of their lives. Fugue states occur when an individual takes physical flight, without conscious knowledge of how he/she got from one location to another.

Dissociation is linked to trauma, particularly when the traumatic situation is ongoing. The more chronic and severe the trauma, the greater the likelihood of extensive dissociation. Lindemann (1944) wrote that "walling off" awareness or memory of the traumatic event is a valuable defense as long as the threat persists. However, as I've mentioned previously, clinicians who work with trauma survivors believe that the trauma must eventually be brought into awareness and put into perspective, or the repressed memories will appear in the form of intrusive thoughts, nightmares, reenactments, or emotional problems.

In my experience, many clinicians observe dissociation in children but remain unsure about how to proceed. Over the years, I have developed the following specific techniques for addressing dissociation:

Develop a language. The first step in addressing dissociation is to develop a way to communicate about it. I ask children about dissociation by saying, "Everybody has times when they're doing something and suddenly they notice that they seem to have gone away in their mind. Like when you're on a long drive and you get bored and you start thinking about different things, and suddenly you got to where you were going and you're surprised. Does that ever happen to you?" The child usually responds positively to the description. I then ask what name they give this process. Children have many names for dissociation, including "spacing out," "getting little," "going inside," "fazing out," and others. Once dissociation is labelled, it can be discussed.

Assess patterns of use. The next step is to inquire when the child dissociates; I ask children to tell me about the last time it happened, or when they think it happens most. As their attention is focused on dissociation, children may notice when they are using this defense.

The clinician and child can review similarities between dissociative experiences. For example in one case, the child seemed to dissociate more when he was alone, and when he was reminded of his father.

Help determine dissociative sequencing. Everyone who uses dissociation as a coping strategy has his/her own unique ways of generating a dissociative response. I find it useful to ask the child to "pretend to dissociate," paying particular attention to the body, emotions, sensations, and thoughts. Once the child is pretending to dissociate, either in the therapy office or at home, I ask the child to notice: what happens to his/her body and what feelings or sensations are experienced; what kinds of feelings he/she has; and what statements he/she might say internally.

The clinician points out the sequence to the child, possibly writing the information on a piece of paper so that the child has a visual representation. This material becomes particularly helpful when the clinician helps the child identify times when he/she might want to choose an alternative response to dissociation. Using the sequence that has been developed with the child's help, the clinician encourages the child to pretend to dissociate, and then stop the dissociation process at different points.

Explain it as adaptive. I always describe dissociation as a helpful defense: "Sometimes when we have a situation that's scary, or when it's too hard to feel our feelings, we 'space out' for a while. It's a really nice thing to be able to do." At the same time, I want to convey a couple of other messages: There are other ways of coping, and the child will feel more in control if a choice can be made about when to dissociate and when to use other strategies.

Understand precipitants. Once the child discusses times when dissociation is a helpful defense, the clinician can document the issues that seem to elicit this flight response. With some children, it appears to be a singular issue such as sexual arousal, physical pain, anger, or longing. For other vulnerable children, the emotions that precipitate the dissociative response may be numerous.

Address the troublesome emotion. Once identified, the emotions or situations that are troublesome to the child must be addressed in the therapy. The child needs to learn coping strategies so that emotions are not avoided or repressed.

One initial technique I've found useful is to externalize the specific emotion. For example, I'll ask the child to draw a picture of anger. Then looking at the picture, I'll ask the child to put words to the picture, and, finally, I'll give the child some open-ended statements such as, "I feel angry when..." "I feel angry because...." "I'm the angriest at..." As the child tolerates the discussion, the frightening emotion is desensitized. On one occasion a child drew a picture of fear, and when I asked what she wanted to do with her picture of fear, she crumpled it up, put it in a wastebasket, and covered the wastebasket with a bunch of pillows. This was her way of symbolically containing her fear, and over the weeks she removed more and more of the pillows until the crumpled-up piece of paper was visible. At that point she grabbed it, announcing "this is little now." She then threw it in the big garbage can outside my office. It was no longer an overwhelming emotion to her. She had learned to tolerate her uncomfortable feelings by talking to me and her father whenever she was worried or scared.

Give alternatives to the flight response. Once the feelings are identified, and the child tolerates open discussion, alternatives can be articulated. "What can you do when you feel sad?" I inquire, always asking for more than one option. "And what else can you do?" I ask after the child responds. If the child runs out of options, the clinician can volunteer other helpful information by role-modeling, "When I feel sad, sometimes I do or say...." I may also mention "Some children I've worked with tell me they feel lots of different ways, and one of those ways is...." It's important to be in contact with the child's caretakers to assure they will respond accordingly to the child.

To summarize, dissociation is an adaptive and useful strategy to defend against frightening memories, sensations, or thoughts that occur in perceived threatening situations. While dissociation is a valuable technique that allows the child to escape immediately when threatened, it can later be a reflexive response that perpetuates feelings of helplessness and continued avoidance of reality. In addition, dissociation can interfere with the child's potential to develop a repertoire of necessary coping behaviors.

The clinician must evaluate the child's use of dissociation, developing techniques for discussing dissociation, making the sequence of dissociation clear, establishing the common patterns of use, and determining common feelings or sensations that precipitate dissociation. *The goal of treatment with dissociation is to help the child feel in control of choosing when he/she dissociates, and knowing the alternatives to dissociation.*

Transfer of Learning

The abused child may grow to trust the therapist and environment sufficiently to experiment with new behaviors. However, unless the child can transfer the behaviors, or discern which behaviors are transferable, the new knowledge can actually become counterproductive.

In working with abused children it is an error to reinforce behaviors that may precipitate attacks at home. For example, one child client was encouraged to ask questions and say how he felt in therapy. The clinician failed to alert the child that the new behavior could be received differently in different settings. When the child was reunited with his natural family, his mother, threatened by her perceived inability to provide information, would slap him each time he asked a question. It was months before a teacher filed a child abuse report and the child could be protected anew.

The therapist needs to help the child understand that some behaviors may provoke different responses in different settings. For example, when working with an abused child who is learning to talk about feelings, the clinician might ask, "How will it be if you tell your mom and dad how you feel?" or "What do you think they will say or do?" It is necessary to keep stressing, "It's OK to tell me about your feelings. Who else can you tell your feelings to?" Eventually, all children learn that people will respond to them differently and adjust their behavior accordingly.

Prevention and Education

All abused children can benefit from learning skills to employ in difficult, frightening, or abusive situations. Allowing the child to anticipate and plan for crises is useful.

Before the child exits therapy, the clinician can spend some time, in an educational mode, teaching the child about child abuse and prevention. I concentrate on a couple of important points: First, that children can say no, try to run away, and get help if someone scares or bothers them and, second, that if anyone asks them to keep a secret that scares or confuses them, they need to tell someone. I always review the child's support system, making sure they understand whom they can contact when they need help. I also convey to the child that he/she never causes someone to abuse him/her and that the abuser always has problems and needs help.

Some of this education can be done in a group setting. If groups are not available, this educational phase can occur within the context of termination of therapy. While some educational programs talk to young children about being "safe, strong, and free," I prefer to use less abstract concepts. I talk to children about the things that make them powerful; since their physical limitations are painfully clear, I concentrate instead on the powers they all possess, including the power to use words, the power to keep or share their thoughts, the power to keep or share their feelings, and the power to keep or share secrets.

Most children, particularly boys, have a tendency to talk about physical power when asked to think what they would do in the future if someone hurt them or did not take good care of them. The children say they will kick, punch, or kill the abuser. But the reality is that children can be easily overpowered, and even though they don't like to see themselves as helpless, the reality is that they are. Because of that, I tend to reinforce the abilities to think, to decide, to choose, to act, to talk, to tell. These are indeed children's powers and can sometimes help to prevent their victimization. Recognizing these powers enhances self-esteem and feelings of competence.

Finally, abused children are vulnerable to feelings of low self-esteem. I spend considerable time helping children identify their strengths, and I validate them consistently. By the time they leave therapy, my child clients should be using positive affirmations, and relying less on external validation. Children who leave therapy must also have some skills in decision making, impulse control, and anger release; hopefully, the children also know what to do when they feel sad or disappointed.

Clinical Examples

Leroy: A Child Traumatized by Severe Parental Neglect

REFERRAL INFORMATION

Leroy was referred for treatment by a placement worker at the Department of Social Services following a dependency petition and placement in foster care owing to severe parental neglect.

SOCIAL/FAMILY HISTORY

Leroy is a 7-year-old black male, the middle child of three brothers. His mother was reportedly psychotic, and there had been a multitude of suspected child neglect reports throughout Leroy's life. He had been in foster care three previous times and had lived in approximately five different states.

Information on Leroy's mother remained sketchy throughout treatment. Reportedly, she had lived most of her life in Mississippi and was one of six children. Her own mother had numerous relationships with men and only two of the children shared the same natural father. Leroy's mother had been a prostitute, a cook, and a waitress and was currently unemployed and "living on the streets." She had a history of psychiatric problems and drug addiction. She had been hospitalized twice and had been unable to sustain a drug-free lifestyle.

The social service agency had reconstructed enough information to present a picture of a very disruptive and inconsistent environment for the children. Although their maternal grandmother had taken care of them some of the time, the children often lived on the streets with their mother.

Six months prior to the referral for treatment, an anonymous report was made to the Police Department of what appeared to be a situation of unattended children in a housing complex. The police entered the studio apartment to find the three children, Leroy, age 7, Adam, age 5, and Alysha, age 4, partially dressed, hungry, scared, and living in an extremely dirty and disheveled large room. The children did not have beds, and it appeared that they huddled together in a corner to stay warm at night. The youngest child, Alysha, was not toilet trained, and the smell of feces and urine permeated the apartment. The children could not say when their mother had left nor how long they had been alone.

After a medical exam Leroy was hospitalized for malnutrition. He was severely dehydrated; it seemed that whenever food was available to the children, Leroy made sure the younger children ate first. He later stated that his mother mostly fed them uncooked spaghetti. Leroy remained in the hospital until his weight increased beyond the dangerous range. His younger brother was placed in a foster home, and since Alysha had tested borderline mentally retarded, she was placed in a specialized foster home. When Leroy was discharged from the hospital, he was very worried about his siblings (apparently he had been their primary caretaker), was worried about his mother (it appeared he had tried to take care of his mother as well), was depressed and anxious, made indiscriminate attachments, and had nightmares and other sleep disturbances. In addition, he was hoarding food; he had been found in the hospital ward attempting to store leftover food from other children's meals.

PRESENTING PROBLEMS

The overriding concern for Leroy was his severe depression. He had long periods of staring out a window from his bed; he did not want to play with the other children. It was very difficult to engage him in conversation: His responses were monosyllabic. He did not seek contact with anyone and never reached out for anything. Even at times when he seemed in obvious physical discomfort, he was unable to ask for assistance, but waited for the call nurse to check in on him. He frequently arose from sleep in an agitated state, apparently having had vivid dreams, which he claimed to forget instantly.

During the week prior to being released from the hospital Leroy's' depressed state had been replaced by hyperalertness and anxiety focusing on alimentation. He would frequently ask when his next meal would be, and he scavenged the unit for treats; some of the nurses began bringing candy bars and fruit from home in an attempt to relieve his anxiety. It was as though his inevitable exit from the hospital had triggered immense anxiety about what would happen next.

Leroy had stopped asking questions about his mother and siblings, apparently resigned to the fact that their future was as uncertain as his. He did not even ask about his foster home and seemed to quietly await the next of a series of placements. This child seemed certain that he had little, if any, control over his life and seemed to acquiesce in silence.

INITIAL CLINICAL IMPRESSIONS

Leroy came to therapy during his first week in a new foster home. The social service agency provided a transportation worker to bring him back and forth to therapy. As he entered my office for the first time, Leroy held the hand of the transportation worker, whom he had just met, and kept his eyes down, moving slowly. To my knowledge he had never been in therapy before. He was very small for his age and seemed to have difficulty walking.

Leroy said hello to me and little else. He seemed cautious, walked slowly, said few words, and had awkward and constricted movements. I greeted him in the waiting room and took the transportation worker and Leroy to look at the playroom, assuring Leroy that the worker would wait for him and would be nearby. This seemed quite irrelevant to him.

In the playroom Leroy seemed uninterested in the toys and in me. He found a soft ball, which he held and squeezed. I sat nearby and talked to him about the playroom: "Kids come here and get to choose what to play with. Sometimes we play and sometimes we talk. I talk to kids about their thoughts and feelings." It was unclear to me if Leroy understood what I said. I asked if there was anything he would like to do. He said no somberly. I said that I sometimes liked to draw with crayons, and I proceeded to take them out and started coloring. As I did I commented, "I like to use lots of colors" and "When you mix red and yellow you get something that looks like orange." I didn't ask him questions or expect a response, and that seemed to give Leroy the freedom to look around. As I sneaked a peek at him he was scanning the environment slowly; he seemed to be taking everything in and recording it for posterity. It was impossible to know what he was thinking or feeling. I kept drawing. Slowly, Leroy got up and walked to the sink. "Is there water here?" he asked. "Well," I responded, "there isn't any water in the room right now, but I can go get some in the bucket." Leroy said, "I want a drink. I'm thirsty." This was the first of countless requests for food or drink. "Oh," I said, "you want water to drink. We can go get some in the kitchen." We walked to the kitchen together, and Leroy reached out for my hand; he seemed to be accustomed to being led around. I held his hand and as we approached the kitchen he noticed the refrigerator. "Is there food in there?" he asked. "Yes Leroy, some of the people who work here keep snacks and lunches in the refrigerator," I explained. "Oh," he remarked. He drank two small cups of water, and we filled up the bucket to take back to the room. As we walked out he asked, "Do you keep snacks in there?" "Sometimes," I said.

Back in the playroom Leroy grabbed the cups and saucers and the teapot. He filled up the teapot and poured tea into the cups, emptying and filling them over and over. Leroy liked to get his hands wet and then dry them. Every now and then he would fill the cup with water and "sneak a drink." I commented, "You fill up the teapot, pour out the tea, sometimes you drink the tea, sometimes you pour it out, and you do it over again." A very small smile seemed to appear as I told him what I had noticed him do. We spoke very little the rest of the session.

I had told Leroy when we first entered the room that a little bell would go off when it was time to leave. He seemed startled when it did ring yet abruptly dropped everything and went to the door. "Leroy," I told him, "I was glad to meet you today, and I will see you next week." He opened the door and we went to the waiting room. He asked the transportation worker if they could still go get a snack, and she quickly said, "Of course, Leroy, I told you we would." He had already extracted a promise from the worker to take care of his anxiety about food, and she left asking him whether MacDonald's or Kentucky Fried Chicken was preferable.

My notes after the first visit were as follows:

This child seems to have difficulty with attachment, as expected. He has a great deal of anxiety about food and eating. His play was focused on water, drinking, filling, and emptying. He asked about the refrigerator downstairs. I want to be careful to give him the space to make choices and experience a sense of control. I will be nondirective and document play themes, attempting to build a therapeutic relationship. I believe trust will be difficult to build. It seems his life has been full of disappointments. Need to check in with his foster parents and need to talk to the transportation worker about not feeding him.

TREATMENT PLANNING

I called the social service agency following my first visit with Leroy. I wanted to develop a treatment plan for this child and wanted to know more about his current status and plan in foster care. The social worker informed me that the mother had never been located after the children were picked up and taken to the hospital. There was speculation that the mother was prostituting again and probably knew the children were in custody. The hospital nurse stated that a black woman had called to ask about the children but had hung up when she was placed on hold. The social service agency had contacted the maternal grandmother, who was ambivalent about caring for the children at this time, particularly without the mother's knowledge. The grandmother matter-of-factly stated that her daughter would show up sooner or later and she hoped it would be later. She said that her daughter's life was hopeless and that she was "no good." "Those children are better off without her," she said, adding, "The good Lord's tired of waiting." The grandmother was curt and uncoopera-tive; it appeared she was accustomed to inquiries about the children, and her frustration resounded loudly.

Long-term placement was planned for Leroy, given the lack of familial resources at the time. The younger children would be released for adoption because they were younger and seen as easier to adopt. If the mother returned to Mis-sissipi or was located locally, attempts would be made to provide services to see if reunification was possible. Given the mother's history, this was unlikely although there had been periods in which she seemed to make reasonable efforts to care for the children. If the mother did not surface after one year, attempts would be made to terminate parental rights for the younger children.

This information helped me structure a treatment plan. Leroy would need some help separating from his siblings, his mother, and his grandmother. Although some initial contact with his siblings might decrease Leroy's anxiety about their well-being, a permanent separation might become inevitable and contact after an adoption might not be feasible. It was also important for me to know that placement with the grandmother was not realistic. Leroy would probably eventually ask about his future—doing so would, in fact, be a good prognostic sign.

I was relieved to hear that the social worker had placed Leroy in a home already structured to provide continuity of care and planned to make contact with Mrs. G., the foster parent, as soon as possible.

BEGINNING PHASE OF TREATMENT

During the next five visits a ritual was clearly established. I would have the bucket full of water and the cups and saucers within reach. Leroy did water play, said little, and seemed to enjoy my verbal observations of his behavior. The fifth week he asked, "Do you have snacks here today?" "No," I said, "I don't." He seemed disappointed. "There's a refrigerator downstairs," he stated.

"Yes, there is, Leroy."

"I want to see it."

"OK, we can walk downstairs." We went downstairs and looked at the refrigerator; Leroy seemed fascinated.

"Lunches are in there."

"Yes," I said, "some lunches are probably in there."

"Can I see?" he asked with wide eyes.

"Yeah, we can open it up," I replied. His eyes were even wider as he stood in front of the open refrigerator for what seemed like an interminable time. He looked at every shelf, every nook and cranny, with his hands by his side. "I have apples at my house," he remarked. "Oh," I said, "you have apples too." "Not me," he corrected, "Mrs. Glennis." "Oh," I repeated, "Mrs. Glennis, your foster mother, has apples." "Yeah," he stated proudly, "her refrigerator is bigger and smells better." "OK," I said, as we went upstairs.

I had Mrs. Glennis come in at about this time. She was a very kind black woman in her 50s. She had been a foster parent for 18 years; she was obviously experienced and concerned for Leroy. "That boy is always eating," she explained. "No matter how much you give him, he always wants more. His eyes are bigger than his stomach. Poor sweetie, just last week I went to his room at night 'cause he was crying. I held him for a long time and rocked him, asking him over and over what was wrong. Finally," she went on, "he said he was thinking about his mama and what she was eating. He told me sometimes his mama did bad things and sometimes the bad men would hurt her and push her down the stairs. That poor child," Mrs. Glennis said, "God only knows what kind of goings on he's seen."

Mrs. Glennis was a single mother and had her two adult children living with her. In addition to Leroy, there were two other foster children, Roshad and Kelya. She said they were all sweet children and got along just fine. The only problem she acknowledged was that the children would fight with Leroy when he stole money from them; they would call him a "fat pig" and make snorting noises at him. Leroy would appear hurt by this and would run to his room and hide.

Mrs. Glennis said that Leroy had improved a lot since first moving in. "He asks me questions now, and he stays out and watches TV with us at night. At first," she remarked, "he would only want to be in his room."

When I asked Mrs. Glennis to describe the routine at home, she said that things were pretty quiet until all the children got home from school. (They all walked to a nearby school together.) She usually had cookies, pies, or cakes waiting for the children, with some milk. "I usually give Leroy a big old piece, 'cause I got to fatten him up." Then the children would do their homework or go out and play while she warmed up dinner. "I usually cook the dinner while they're in school and have everything ready for them when they get home." After dinner, which she described as "quiet," the children would watch TV or play a game and then she would get them ready for bed. They would take a bath or shower, put out their clothes for the next day, and say their prayers. Sometimes, she reported, Leroy would eat a little piece of something that he had saved up before going to sleep.

Mrs. Glennis said she had few disciplinary problems with the children. "I used to get rowdy kids, but now I've told Mrs. Calbot that I can only handle the quiet children." She said, "They know when I'm mad. I just got to look their way and they behave. They don't want me mad. Just as quiet as I can be is as loud as I am when I'm mad."

When asked about other things she noticed about Leroy, Mrs. Glennis stated that he seemed "a little strange sometimes." When I asked her to elaborate she said, "Well, sometimes you'll be talking with him and he seems to look like through you, like you weren't even there. Sometimes," she goes on, "when he's watching TV, he just sucks his thumb and seems to be in another world. He does cry more than the other two, and when they call him a 'crybaby,' he usually goes to his room and falls asleep. If he gets really mad he tells the others that they are not his real brother and sister and that he has a real brother and sister that are better than them. When the kids didn't believe him, he came running and almost dragged me out to make sure they knew he was telling the truth."

Mrs. Glennis also announced, with some discomfort, that Leroy "touches himself down there a lot" and that he's very shy about anybody seeing his body. When I asked what she does with his masturbatory behavior, she replied, "I slap his hands...not hard, just so he knows that touching isn't something I want to see." Mrs. Glennis volunteered that she thought it might be good for Leroy to see his brother and sister and stated that she knew the foster mother who was keeping the children. This contact had certainly crossed my mind as well.

I thanked Mrs. Glennis for all her insights. She was providing a structured environment for Leroy, and he was clearly responding in a positive light. I told her that instead of slapping Leroy she might want to try giving him a ball or something to do with his hands since children this age tend to masturbate when they are tired or bored. She agreed to try. In addition, I talked to Mrs. Glennis about Leroy's anxiety about food. "I agree with you that he's had a very difficult life so far," I began. "As you know, he could have died from the severe malnutrition he had. I think now he's extremely worried about getting enough food. At the same time, I worry that if people overfeed him, he might not have a chance to learn to deal with his anxiety." Mrs. Glennis seemed a little offended since she commented that she wasn't overfeeding the child but only making sure "he got some meat on his bones." I told her I also wanted to see Leroy have good physical health and encouraged her to try from time to time, when she thought of it, to either say no to his request for more food or tell him that if he was still hungry in an hour, he could have more then. She did not seem as responsive to this suggestion as she was to the one about the masturbatory behavior.

I contacted Leroy's teacher to ask about his school behavior and discovered that he was doing fairly well in the first grade. An initial educational assessment had found his verbal and math skills almost nonexistent, and the social service agency had been unable to locate any prior school records. The teacher said that Leroy was very compliant in class. "Sometimes," she declared, "you forget he's here." She also mentioned his obsession with food and had noticed his scavenging through trash cans during recess. She had also seen him hide food in his backpack to take home. Some of the children had ridiculed him for this and, like his foster siblings, labeled him a "hog" and a "pig." Academically, Leroy was catching up nicely and seemed to be proud when he earned a star or a happy face on his work. The teacher said she saw no behavioral or unexpected academic problems at this time, but saw Leroy as staying a little on the periphery socially. "I encourage him to play team sports or try group projects, but he prefers to be by himself." The only other comment was that Leroy had taken a liking to an assistant teacher and always looked forward to seeing her.

After seeing Leroy for ten more sessions (2½ months), I saw several clear patterns. Leroy's play was ritualistic, and he seemed to be reenacting his own deprivation and alimentation. He was obsessed with getting enough of everything. He had begun to pay close attention to setting the time and would frequently say, "you set it on 48 minutes, not 50." On several occasions he asked whether I had snacks in the refrigerator. Using my nondirective approach, I would always answer, "You like to know whether or not I have food in the refrigerator." "Well, do you?" he demanded once. I answered, "Nope, not today." The refrigerator in my office had become symbolic of food he could not access, and although he was not yet comfortable to ask for food, or take food, he almost always commented on the refrigerator.

During this time I always gave Leroy ample choice of activities. Only once or twice did he want to color, and he always turned to the same page, noting that "no one else" colored on his page. He was meticulous about coloring inside the lines. From time to time Leroy appeared glad to come into the playroom, even rushing in. On one occasion when I was 5 minutes late, he immediately asked if he would still have his whole time. I told him of course he would. This was his first broad, although brief, smile.

Treatment Plan

My treatment plan for Leroy was outlined in the third month and was documented in my records as follows:

1. Individual nondirective play therapy with Leroy
   a. Document play themes and patterns; note symbols used in play.
   b. Observe and remain nonintrusive.
   c. Encourage choice and a feeling of control.
   d. Increase therapy to twice weekly.
2. Interactional issues
   a. Observe level of interaction initiated by L.
   b. Observe interactional play with toys/dolls.
   c. Obtain information on ongoing interactions with foster mother, foster siblings, teacher, assistant teacher, and peers.
   d. Define level of interaction with therapist: number of questions asked, number of "I" statements, number of spontaneous comments.
   e. Encourage L.'s meeting his own needs, i.e., asking to do something, demanding his time, etc.
3. Trauma work
   a. Be attuned to symbols of trauma of malnutrition, and separation from mother; watch for post-traumatic play.

b. Become directive if material does not deepen over time.

4. Coordination

   a. Keep in touch with social worker; submit reports as required.

   b. Meet with foster mother at least once a month and gauge progress in home (check on overfeeding). Also, check on quality of attachment, anxious behaviors, and nightmares.

   c. Attempt to have some contact initiated between Leroy and his biological brother and sister.

MIDDLE PHASE OF TREATMENT

Meeting with Leroy twice a week was very successful. He began to make an appropriate attachment to me and deepened his therapeutic work tremendously. His play shifted dramatically 2 months after beginning his biweekly sessions. He stopped playing with the cups and saucers and turned his attention to an array of baby bottles on display. I am sure he had always noticed these, but now he abruptly began to gather them up, fill them with water, and empty them. His affect changed during these filling and emptying sessions. He would breathe hard, become physically still, and check with me frequently and nervously. Then one day, as if mustering up all his strength, he put the nipple of the baby bottle in his mouth and looked at me. I made eye contact with him, and he did not look away. "You're drinking from the baby bottle," I said. He walked slowly to a stack of pillows, and lay down on them, and sucked vigorously on the bottle. When he finished all the water, the bottle fell from his mouth. "More," he said quietly. "You want to drink more from the baby bottle," I said. I took the bottle, filled it up with water, and gave it back to him. I went back to my seat next to the water tray. Leroy lay with his legs curled up, on his side, sucking on the nipple. He was no longer sucking hard, he was suckling quietly. The bell of the timer disturbed him, and he seemed angry that he had to get up. He threw the bottle across the room and walked out the door. "Leroy," I shouted, "let me say good-bye to you." I crouched down so that we could make eye contact, and I said, "You had a lot to drink from the baby bottles. You threw the bottle away when the bell rang. You might have liked to stay and drink a little longer. The bottles will be here next time you come. I'll see you then, Leroy." He walked away; as he grabbed the transportation worker's hand, he looked back at me and waved.

Leroy was shy when he came the next time; he may have been embarrassed by his sucking on the baby bottle. He drew for a while, and I took the opportunity to ask him to draw a picture of himself. "What do you mean?" he asked. "Well, just draw a picture of you," I said. Figure 1 is Leroy's first drawing of himself. When I asked him to draw a picture of his family, he drew Figure 2. It is striking to see how large he seems in the picture and how overwhelmed by the inconsistent and

FIGURE 1

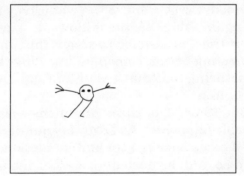

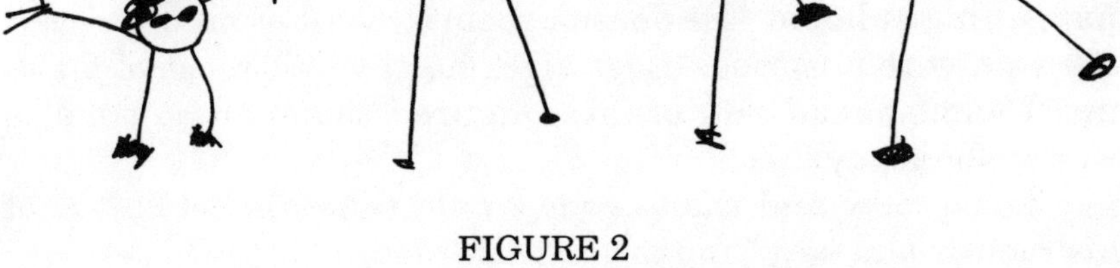

FIGURE 2

barren environment. His drawing is typical of drawings produced by much younger children. In the drawing of a child of Leroy's age and background, the lack of body is probably symbolic of his lack of body image, due to his being so severely malnourished, so developmentally delayed, and, now, so physically uncomfortable with his predictable weight gain. The family picture reflects his sense of isolation. None of the family members has a mouth, and the mother's small size indicates Leroy's view of himself as the caretaker.

While drawing his family Leroy stated, "I love my mom. She's a nice mom. She's not bad." It was almost as if he were reassuring himself rather than being self-revealing. "You have a nice mom and you love her," I repeated. Before I could say, "She's not bad," Leroy asserted, "AND SHE'S NOT BAD!" I agreed, "That's right, Leroy, she's not a bad mommy. You miss her," I added. Leroy went to the water tray to fill up his bottles once again, then to the pillows to suckle quietly. Unlike the first time, he seemed to accept the time limitation and to get up feeling better, somehow, knowing that he could control his nurturing and that I would fill up his bottle and bring it back to him.

After about 10 or 12 of these nurturing sessions, something remarkable happened. As Leroy lay quietly I heard him say, "Eliana." I came over to him and he motioned for me to sit down. I did so, and he curled up so that his head was on my lap; he lay comfortably and finished his bottle. As he left that day he waved, then turned away.

Another month and a half followed of these nurturing sessions. Sometimes Leroy would reach over and hold my hand. Once he took my hand and put it on his head. Instinctively, I stroked his head, and he fell asleep. He woke up to the bell, apparently feeling nurtured. He was leaving these sessions looking less anxious and somewhat happier. Mrs. Glennis called me to tell me that something different was happening at home. "He doesn't seem to want as much to eat," she said with surprise. "Last night he gave his piece of pie to me. I went ahead and ate it; I figured this was no time to worry about my diet."

Every now and then Leroy would take his bottle out of his mouth and say, "You are not my mom."

"No, Leroy, I am not your mom."

"My mom's name is Loretta."

"Yes, Leroy, your mom's name is Loretta."

Then he would resume the suckling behaviors feeling reassured. These statements seemed to be a sign that Leroy was functioning in the real world and developing coping strategies. This real world was one of feelings: he longed for his mother's nurturing, yet he faced the reality of her limitations. His mother was an unrewarding and inconsistent object. He would need to rely on others and, eventually, himself for emotional nurturance. He had found a way to deal with his longing, and he seemed to be repairing himself through this enactive play.

Every other week or so, Leroy stopped his nurturing sessions. He would draw or build structures with building blocks: Eventually, he ventured over to the dollhouse. At first, he sat in front of the dollhouse and seemed to look inside, afraid to move anything. I commented, "You sit quietly looking inside the house. You don't touch anything. You sit outside, looking in." I brought out the small family figures that could be used inside the dollhouse. (Leroy had always avoided the shelf with human figures. His play until now had always been with objects: blocks, crayons, even some trucks and small cars that he drove around in circles.) He looked at me surprised. This was the first time I had chosen something for him to play with. "Is this their house?" he asked. "It could be," I replied. I looked at the house and he looked at the dolls. He grabbed the mother doll and put her in the kitchen. "She cooks," he stated firmly. "The lady is in the kitchen cooking." He moved away quickly and drew for the rest of the session. He had learned some songs from his foster mother and delighted in singing while he drew. I would always tell him, "You sing pretty songs, Leroy; you remember all the words and the tunes that go with them." He seemed to feel proud, and over the weeks his voice was becoming stronger. He would smile broadly when he finished his songs; I would smile back. Leroy took my hand as we walked out of the play sessions. He had had many transportation workers, and he no longer took their hands as he left; he now walked beside them, seemingly confident.

Eight months of therapy had transpired, and Leroy's progress was tremendous. He had finished one full term in the same school, and his grades had improved. (On one occasion, Leroy ran into the waiting room anxious to see me. He boasted appropriately that he had gotten an A in writing. "Mrs. Esther is going to make me my own pie," he announced.) One area reminiscent of Leroy's malnutrition persisted. Mrs. Glennis's attempts to stop overfeeding him had been marginal at best. She would frequently tell me that, try as she might, she could not say no to Leroy's requests for extra food. Mrs. Glennis was an obese woman, and her natural children were obese as well. It appeared that she was convinced that children should be very round; it was difficult to combat her established belief system. She had continued to reward Leroy with food, and Leroy still responded to this type of reward.

In therapy some headway was made in helping Leroy cope with his anxiety about not getting enough food. He had continued to ask about the refrigerator downstairs and would frequently ask to look at what was inside; he would remark about what he liked and what he didn't like. Usually, the conversation ended with his assertion that Mrs. Glennis's refrigerator had "bigger and better" things than ours did.

I had purchased a toy refrigerator and toy foods for the playroom. Leroy had noticed them immediately; he played with them by taking the foods out, counting them, and putting them back. Other children played with the toys, a fact that Leroy had never overlooked. Leroy's play seemed to be an attempt to verify that no one had taken any of the foods. "Do other kids come here to play?"

"You want to know if other kids come here to play. Yes, they do Leroy."

"Do you come here with other kids?"

"You want to know if I come to the playroom with other children. Yes, Leroy, sometimes I come to the playroom with other children," I replied. There followed countless questions about the other children and their therapy. The foods were recounted every week; eventually, some turned up missing.

Leroy was surprised and worried. He looked everywhere for the missing items. When he couldn't find them he withdrew into a corner. "Those kids are bad to steal things," he concluded.

"You really don't like it when you've left things in their place and they are missing," I said.

"Will you get new ones?"

"I don't know, Leroy."

"Well, you should."

"You really like it when things stay the same. You don't like it when things disappear." We were now talking about his mother. "I don't want to play with that anyway," he announced. Thus he rejected the very toy that caused him consternation. He would return to it eventually. "You have feelings about things you miss," I observed.

Two weeks after this session Leroy asked to write a letter to his mother. "Sure, Leroy. You can write a letter to your mom," I said. In his best "A" handwriting he wrote, "I love you Mom." "Send it to my mom," he said as he walked away. "You want your mom to get this letter saying you love her," I said. "Will you send it?" he asked. I was stumped but replied, "Next time you come we'll send it together." I needed some time to think this through.

The following week Leroy didn't mention the letter. When he said he wanted to stop coloring, I said, "Last week you wanted to send this letter to your mom. Here's an envelope." We put his mother's name on the envelope. "I don't know an address for your mom, Leroy. What shall we put?" I asked. "Put Mississippi," he said. "OK," I agreed. We took the letter to the mailbox, and Leroy could barely reach to insert it in the box. "God will take it to her," he announced. "OK," I said. "You really want her to know you love her." No mention was made of a reply. Several months later Leroy wanted to write a letter from his mother to him. He wrote, "I love you, Mom." He wanted to walk to the mailbox again. This time the envelope did have an address: Mrs. Glennis's address. Leroy brought the letter in happily. "It came today," he announced. "I got my letter from Mom." He saved that letter in his room.

TERMINATION

The social worker called one day and announced that Leroy would be sent to Mississippi in the next few weeks. She stated that Leroy's mother had been arrested and released to her mother's care. The maternal grandmother had agreed to let her live in the family home as long as she had a job. Leroy and his brother were to be returned to Mississippi, where a reunification plan would begin. I was stunned and concerned about the abrupt way in which termination would occur. Leroy had made great strides: He had formed an attachment with his foster mother, had done well in school and in therapy, and had begun to feel secure in his environment. With one phone call, this was all disrupted. I saw Leroy immediately to tell him that he would be moved back to his mother in Mississippi. He looked away quietly. "Will Adam and Alysha come too?" he asked. "I think so, Leroy, but we'll have to check with Mrs. Calbot [the social worker]," I replied. Since the mother had been located within the 1-year time frame, it was possible that termination of parental rights would be deferred. Leroy asked where he would live and when he had to go. I responded, "I think you'll be with your grandma but, again, we'll talk together to Mrs. Calbot; you should be leaving in about a week and a half. We'll be able to meet three more times." Leroy appeared somber and began to color quietly in the corner. "I'm going to miss you, Leroy," I said. He continued his coloring. "It's hard to say good-bye to people you like," I told him. "I like you," he said spontaneously. "I like you too," I said.

The following session I brought a scrapbook and a Polaroid camera. I told Leroy that today would be special because I was going to take some pictures for him that he could take to Mississippi with him. I took pictures of the playroom, the sink he played with initially, the baby bottles (he wanted me to take a picture of him with the bottle on the pillow he used to lay on), and a picture of the building from the outside. He took a few pictures of me in the playroom, and one of the staff took a picture of us together. We went to his school, and we took pictures of his classroom and his teacher. We then went to his foster home and took pictures of Mrs. Glennis with Leroy, and of Leroy and the other children. He had a bittersweet smile in most of the pictures, and he carefully placed them on the pages. "I have lots of pictures," he said happily. "Yes, you do," I agreed. "Can I take this with me on the plane?" he asked. "Yes, you can Leroy. You can look at this whenever you want and remember what it was like when you lived in California," I told him. "I like California," he said, "and I like Mississippi."

In our last two sessions we talked about his leaving, saying good-bye, writing letters, and the people and things he would miss in California. He brought the scrapbook to each session and made some drawings inside. He also showed me the other mementos he had included. There were ticket stubs from the movies, his report cards, some homework with stars and happy faces, and some candy bar wrappers. Each session I helped him say good-bye to the playroom and the toys he had played with—but Leroy didn't touch the bottles. It was almost as if he were unable to say good-bye to them.

The last session I gave Leroy a going-away present; he opened it with anticipation. It was a brand-new baby bottle, small enough to be unobtrusive. On the card I had written the following:

Dear Leroy:

I will think of you in Mississippi with your mother, grandmother, and brother and sister. I know that people are helping your mom so she learns how to keep you safe and feed you well. When you look at this little bottle I hope you will remember how you learned to feed yourself and make yourself feel better inside. If you ever feel hungry for food, be sure you talk to your grandmother or teacher. If you ever feel hungry for love, ask a grown-up you trust for a hug or kiss or close your eyes and remember the way you learned to make yourself feel better. I will think of you and remember you always.

Eliana

"This one is just mine?" he asked incredulously. "Just for you," I said. He hugged me spontaneously clutching his little bottle.

DISCUSSION

Leroy was a youngster traumatized by severe parental neglect. He had experienced a chronic sense of helplessness and coped with inconsistent care, separations, relocations, and danger with a sense of resignation. His mother had been drug-dependent for years and had a chaotic lifestyle. Like many victims of malnutrition, Leroy had developed anxiety about getting enough to eat, manifested by his attempts to scavenge for and hoard food. He was lethargic, slept a great deal, and seemed to avoid interpersonal contact. It appeared that Leroy was the primary caretaker for his two younger siblings—and probably for his mother as well. Leroy's presenting problem was depression. Underlying problems included learned helplessness, making indiscriminate attachments, anxiety about his nutritional needs, nightmares, and interactional problems.

In therapy, I decided to use the nondirective approach in an attempt to give Leroy a sense of self-control. I wanted him to make choices, to ask for things, to try to get his own needs met. I wanted him to experience and cope with the anxiety of forming a relationship with me. In time, he would face his fear of and wish for dependency and consistency.

I provided Leroy with play materials that would help him reenact the underlying primary issues of fear, deprivation, and longing. Materials such as cups and saucers, water, baby bottles, a supermarket cart, a refrigerator, and toy food became very significant to Leroy. In addition, he was eventually able to overcome the discomfort they generated and to use the dollhouse and family dolls to act out some of his fantasies about family life. Leroy's perception of houses and homes was somewhat distorted by his experiences: He had moved constantly and had frequently slept huddled on sidewalks.

Leroy's play themes consistently reflected his appropriate preoccupation with nurturing: He was always emptying and filling objects. He symbolized his need for physical nurturance by drinking out of the baby bottles during the sessions and his need for emotional nurturance by suckling on the bottle while lying curled up on the pillows.

Leroy's interactions improved significantly during treatment. He was able to ask questions, direct my participation in the play, and attempt to get his needs met. It was obvious that the therapy became important to him and that he looked forward to coming to therapy. He always made sure he set the timer to the exact time, and he respected the limits imposed. He learned to deal with the anxiety of not eating during our sessions while knowing that there was food in the building. He was also able to tolerate the fact that other children played with "his" (toy) food.

Leroy learned to self-nurture during the treatment. He satisfied primitive urges to suckle, got more to drink when he wanted, and directed me to make physical contact with him during some of his reenactments all the while successfully differentiating between reality and fantasy, his mother and me. Through fantasy he was able to compensate for his early experiences of deprivation. He stopped making indiscriminate attachments and remained polite but distant with new transportation workers. He made an important attachment to his foster mother, feeling secure and loved in the foster home environment; at the same time, he seemed to have an internal restriction, understanding full well that foster care is temporary and can be changed abruptly.

I used directive play minimally with Leroy; I guided his involvement in the dollhouse play, perceiving his ambivalence. Had he avoided play when I brought the dolls out, I would have noted this response, and allowed him to choose what to do next.

Unfortunately, termination was premature and abrupt. Under the circumstances, I thought it best to prepare Leroy to leave in a structured way. He had made tremendous strides and had some skills he could use in the future, which would surely be uncertain at best. It was difficult to reassure him about how things would be. The social worker assured us both that she would make a comprehensive transfer of material, including my termination summary. She was also determined to make sure that his therapy continued in Mississippi. Leroy went back to his mother stronger and a little more self-defined and confident.

Johnny: A Child Traumatized by Sexual Abuse

REFERRAL INFORMATION

Johnny was referred for treatment by a Child Protective Services worker after an allegation of sexual abuse by an unrelated male adult who boarded with the paternal grandmother at the same time that Johnny and his mother lived with her.

SOCIAL/FAMILY HISTORY

Johnny was nearly 5 years old at the time of the referral. He was the only child of David and Maggie, who had divorced shortly after his birth. David had been violent with both mother and child and all ties between natural father and child were severed at the time of the divorce. Maggie had fled with Johnny to her mother-in-law, who had offered shelter. Maggie's own mother and father had died in a car accident when she was 11; she then had lived in a number of foster homes and had lived two years in a group home prior to reaching majority age. It was during her stay at the group home that Maggie had met David and become pregnant. Their first child was stillborn, and Johnny was conceived two years later.

David was the oldest of five brothers. He had been a ward of the court since the age of 14, when he stole a car and drove it across the state line to sell. David had spent most of his adolescence in juvenile detention and group homes; he had a long-standing drug-dependency problem.

Maggie called Child Protective Services (CPS) when Johnny told her that Larry, the boarder, was hurting him. Johnny told CPS that Larry had "hurt his bottom." A medical exam revealed positive findings for a sexually transmitted disease. Larry had fled upon learning that Johnny had been taken to the doctor; the police found him, placed him under arrest, and held him for a hearing. Johnny's paternal grandmother was incredulous about Larry's involvement in molesting the child. She knew Larry's parents and refused to believe Johnny, seeing him as confused. She questioned Johnny relentlessly, encouraging him to say that it was "someone else" who had hurt him and that he had never been alone with Larry. In spite of the grandmother's incredulity, the district attorney charged Larry with lewd and lascivious conduct with a minor under the age of 14, and a preliminary hearing ensued. The district attorney had prepared Johnny to testify, and it appeared the boy would be able to testify about the abuse in a clear enough fashion.

At the preliminary hearing Johnny was articulate enough to state that Larry had "hurt his bottom." Upon cross-examination he was asked, "What did you do when Larry hurt you?"; Johnny replied, "I stabbed Larry's eyes, broke his knees, and pushed him off a mountain." Johnny's case was dismissed because he was not seen as a credible witness even though there were medical findings conclusive of sexual abuse. There was little doubt that something sexual had happened to the child, but it was difficult to ascertain exactly what it was and who the perpetrator was.

Johnny had an array of problem behaviors. He had nightmares and clung to his mother. He was suddenly frightened of noises, new people, and of being alone. His mother and caretakers were concerned with his excessive masturbation, his aggression, and his constant preoccupation with the devil. Mother and paternal grandmother had both been perplexed by the latter; they denied ever teaching Johnny anything about the devil.

Because Johnny's grandmother had refused to believe his allegations against Larry, Maggie moved out of her house and relocated in a nearby county. It was after this move that she and Johnny were referred to me for treatment.

CLINICAL IMPRESSIONS

Johnny was a very attractive but disruptive 5-year old. He was articulate and bright but unresponsive to limits and found it difficult to contain his curiosity. When he entered the office, his agitation elicited everyone's attention. He opened doors into other therapists' offices, drank numerous cups of water, crumpling up the cups and throwing them everywhere, climbed the chairs, turned the music up, tried to take fish out of a fish tank in the waiting room, and generally created chaos.

Johnny's mother was ineffective and inconsistent. She seemed mortified by his behavior and was alternately threatening, helpless, and solicitous. She asserted that Johnny's "terrible behavior" was new and had appeared after he was molested by Larry. Prior to the molestation, she noted, Johnny had been quiet and obedient. Mother was very eager to have her son receive some help and to receive guidance and support for herself as well.

The first few sessions Johnny entered and exited the playroom every few minutes. He didn't seem able to tolerate being alone with me. When he went to the waiting room to verify his mother's presence, he usually did something to elicit her concern, such as climb and fall, push the hot water lever on the water fountain, or tear up some brochures in the waiting room.

I quickly began to set limits. "Johnny, look. This is a timer. We have 50 minutes together, and when the bell rings it's time to leave," I told him. "Let me see that," he said, grabbing the clock and resetting it. The third time he grabbed it I put it up high and told him, "This timer stays here during our sessions." He got mad at me and went running to his mother. I came out and offered him my hand, saying "Come and see the toys I have in my playroom." He would not take my hand, yet he followed me as I turned my back and went to the playroom.

The first two meetings I could not contain him. He took down every toy from the shelves without looking at them. He threw the toys down, scattering them all over the room. At one point I said, "Johnny, the toys all have a place on the shelves. Let's put them back." "No," he said decisively as he ran out of the room.

It occurred to me that Johnny might want the door open. Sometime during the end of the second session, I said, "Let's leave the door a little bit open; that way you can look out and know that you can leave if you really want." He responded very well to the door being ajar and sat down to color. When I asked him what his drawing was about, he yelled loudly, "It's Larry, stupid." "What's he doing?" I asked. Johnny left the room. By the third session he stayed in the playroom with few interruptions. Every now and then he would take something out to his mother or ask to go to the bathroom.

Johnny had a short attention span. He changed from one toy or type of play to another every 6 minutes or so. "Put this back, stupid," he would say, handing me the toy he no longer wanted. I put the toys back and noted that he had begun to create a structure around his play, organizing a beginning, a middle, and an end.

I met with Johnny's mother weekly. She described Johnny's obsessive articulation about Larry and the devil. She noted that this behavior exacerbated at nighttime; Johnny was afraid to go to sleep, and bedtime was now the center for conflict. Johnny wanted the light on and the door open and came to her bedroom five to ten times a night.

About the third session I asked Johnny about his dreams: "What happens after you go to sleep at night?" He looked at me with wide eyes and spoke quietly: "The devil comes to take me to his bosom."

"What's the devil look like?"

"He's red with horns."

"You know, Johnny, I have a little doll that looks like the devil."

"No you don't," he challenged.

"Would you like to see it?"

"No." He seemed afraid.

"That's fine, Johnny. Here's a piece of paper. Draw me a picture of the devil that comes at night."

Johnny took the paper and drew a picture bright with reds and blacks (Figure 1). He was very purposeful as he chose the colors for his devil picture, closing his eyes in apparent deep concentration. When the picture was complete, he rushed out to show it to his mother. "Mom, Mom, this is the devil that comes in the nighttime. Eliana has a devil too." I explained to the mother and Johnny that I had

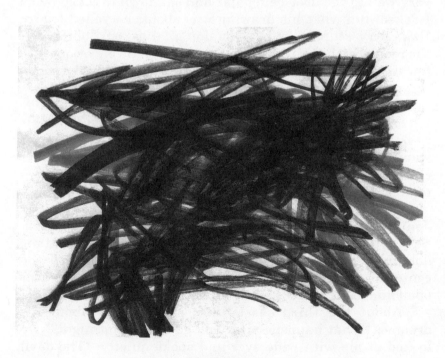

FIGURE 1

a small figure of the devil in the playroom; I said that Johnny and I had been talking about his scary dreams. Johnny spontaneously said, "The devil has powers. He'll kill you too." I kneeled down so I could make eye contact, looked at him, and said, "Johnny, I know someone has talked to you a lot about the devil and how scary he can be. I want you to know that God protects us from the devil, and God will take good care of you and your mommy now." "No, he won't," he said. "God doesn't like bad children." I decided to be assertive and stated firmly, "God loves good and bad children just the same. God understands that the devil scares kids and makes kids think they're bad. You and I will talk more and ask God to help us fight off the devil, OK?" Johnny grabbed his mother's hand, saying, "Let's go, Mom."

The next time he came Johnny again emphasized, "God doesn't love bad children."

"What do you do that's bad?"

"Nothing," Johnny answered, "but I do bad things to Larry."

"What bad things do you do?"

"I can't tell you."

"What will happen if you tell?"

"Larry will kill us."

"Who will Larry kill?"

"Me and my mommy."

"Did Larry tell you that?" I asked. He nodded yes. "You know what Johnny?"

"Huh?"

"Larry is gone now. He won't hurt you or your mom. He lives somewhere far away now, and he doesn't know where you live."

"Yes he does."

"I don't think so," I said calmly.

"Your mom hasn't told anybody where you live so you can be very, very safe."

"Larry can find us," Johnny said sadly.

"You're really scared of Larry."

"He hurts me."

"How does he do that?"

"He puts a stick in my bottom."

"He's wrong to do that. Grown-ups shouldn't hurt kids like that."

"Kids are stupid," Johnny responded.

"Why, Johnny, why are kids stupid?"

"Because they can't make the bad things stop."

"Kids aren't stupid, Johnny. They're just little, and they can't fight great big mean people." Johnny looked despondent. "Look, Johnny," I said as I grabbed a large and a small cloth doll. "This is you and this is Larry. What's the difference?"

Johnny started beating the big "Larry" doll with his fist, saying, "He's big and tall. He has a beard."

"That's right. The grown-up man is big and tall. The kid is little."

"He's bad," Johnny added.

"Yes, Johnny, when he puts a stick in your bottom and hurts you, he's doing bad things."

"Yeah," he repeated, now turning the male doll over and hitting the doll's buttocks with his fist.

"Is the kid bad?" I asked.

"Yeah, he's bad too."

"How come? What makes him bad?"

"I don't know," Johnny said as he kicked both dolls away. "How much time do we have left?"

"Oh, about 25 minutes."

"I want to make some cookies with clay."

"Sounds good to me," I said. "We talked about Larry, the devil, and scary things for a long time. We can make cookies now."

Johnny came to the next session with a pressing question. "Where is God?" he asked. "People say God is everywhere, watching over us," I stated. I made a mental note to ask his mother about her religious beliefs and if and how she had explained the concept of God to Johnny. He immediately asked what God looked like. I told him everyone had a different picture of God in his or her mind, and maybe he could draw a picture of what *he* thought God might look like. Johnny thought for a long while before choosing the yellow crayon and making a large yellow ball that filled the page. He then made a smile. Eyes were notably missing (Figure 2).

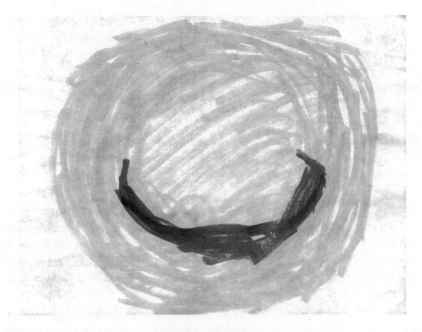

FIGURE 2

"God is strong and big," he said in a steady voice. "Yes, Johnny, he is," I agreed. "He can't beat up the devil," Johnny said, adding in a soft voice, "maybe sometimes."

I once again talked about nighttime dreams. "Remember you told me the devil comes after you go to sleep." "Yeah," Johnny replied. "Maybe you can keep your picture of God under the pillow and the devil might not want to come around so much," I suggested. Johnny seemed intrigued by this idea, yet he appeared troubled as well. "What are you thinking?" I asked. "I want to make a copy on the machine," he replied. Johnny had been very interested in the photocopy machine, and I had shown him how it worked. When he made his pictures, he would sometimes leave the original in my office and take a copy home with him. It was clear that he wanted to leave a copy of his God picture in the playroom. He also made a second copy for the secretary, stating, "God is everywhere. This is what God looks like." She had thanked him and put the picture on the wall.

His mother reported that Johnny's nightmares had decreased and that his devil talk was now usually concluded with a discussion of God and God's powers. She said that Johnny had stated that he wasn't really bad, that the devil might have tricked him. "God knows I'm really good," he had told his mother; she had agreed.

These themes of good and bad, devil and God, and being watched and protected by God continued over time. Johnny had periods of greater or lesser concern, and I asked his mother to monitor his TV and movie watching. Scary movies on TV usually caused regression: His insomnia and night terrors resurfaced. I also asked his mother to keep her conversations about Larry out of Johnny's earshot (she would sometimes become agitated talking to friends about what had happened to her son and how her mother-in-law hadn't believed him and how the courts had failed to prosecute Larry.)

I turned my attention to Johnny's ongoing aggressive behavior. He had continued to exhibit aggressive behavior with children he knew and had been expelled from his preschool after a number of suspensions. His mother had taken Johnny to four child-care workers, all of whom refused to keep him, citing his relentlessly cruel treatment of other children. Johnny was reportedly hitting, biting, kicking, pushing, and yelling at peers; varied attempts to curb his behavior had failed.

I raised the question directly with Johnny. "I hear that you can't go back to Mrs. Jenkins's school anymore. How come?" Johnny stated that his teacher was mean, the kids were stupid, and he didn't like it there anyway. I asked again what had happened that made Mrs. Jenkins ask him to leave.

Finally, he said, "I'm bad to the other kids."

"What do you do or say that's bad," I inquired. And he honestly stated that he hit kids and hurt them. "Why do you think you do that?"

"I don't know. I just want to."

"What do you think about it after you do it?"

"Nothing. Just...well, I'm bad."

"You know, Johnny, I want to help you stop hurting other kids. Do you think we can work together on that?"

"I don't know," he again answered honestly.

My hypothesis was that Johnny's aggression reflected the following: He was manifesting anxiety about being hurt and helpless; he was feeling potentially threatened in his caretaking environment; and he was still struggling with his confusion about good and bad: Bad people were powerful, good people were weak and defenseless. He would usually only attack bigger boys. When he elicited negative attention and was punished for his badness, he might also have been asking for limits on his bad behavior.

My first intervention was to talk with Johnny about good and bad power. I explained that it was OK to be and to feel powerful and strong. I specified that some people used power in a good way and others used power in a bad way. I asked him to help me come up with good and bad ways to show power. Bad ways were clear to him. He listed the following: "making people do what you want; hitting people; pushing people around; biting people; kicking a dog; having millions of dollars because then people do what you want." He couldn't think of any ways to use power in a good way. When I asked him to think about ways that being strong could help, he arrived at, "carrying heavy things." I agreed. He then got up and tried to lift a heavy box. "I'm really strong," he said. "I can see that," I remarked as he carried the box out of the room to show his mother. I told her, "This is a way that Johnny can use his power in a good way." She smiled, understanding my meaning.

In the next few sessions I kept reminding Johnny about good ways to use power. In fact, in one session we talked about the kinds of power children have. "They can punch people out," said Johnny.

"Yeah," I noted, "but littler kids can't punch out bigger kids."

"Sometimes they can."

"Yeah, sometimes, but when it comes to punching out, sometimes you win, sometimes you lose. Think about the kind of power no one can take away."

Johnny drew, raced toy cars, and just before leaving he said, "I know...I know...if I don't want to tell you something, you can't make me."

"That's right, that's a power you have. You have the power to keep your thoughts to yourself."

Once we had established this, Johnny came up with a number of powers children have, including the power to have their own thoughts, their own feelings, to use their own words, to make choices, to go to sleep or stay awake. It was interesting to note that when we talked about choices, Johnny said "I can hit somebody or kick them." I added, "Yeah, and you can hit somebody or *not* hit somebody."

Johnny's mother told me that the child-care worker had called to describe a few altercations with Johnny and had reported that, overall, Johnny was doing better and seemed to be making an effort to do as he was told and avoid fights.

I brought BOBO, a punching bag clown, to the playroom. It was not necessary to explain its use to Johnny. He immediately delighted in hitting it and letting it bounce back for yet another punch. He was tireless; the first time he saw the bag, he spent his entire 50 minutes punching it. The punching had a random quality. Two weeks later, an opportunity arose to alter this type of random release. Johnny came in after having had a fight with a boy at his day-care center. "He makes me mad," he said, charging into the playroom. "I hate him."

"What does he say or do that makes you feel that way?"

"He pushes me around...he thinks he's so tough."

"What did you do with those feelings?"

"I hit him hard."

I pulled out the bag and asked him to pretend this was the little boy and show him how he felt. He socked him with a vengeance. Then I stopped him, asking, "Now put words to your punch. If you were using your words instead of your punch what would you say to him?" He instinctively made fists and took some punches. "Don't use your hands," I directed; "hold your hands together and *think* about punching Stevie out. What would you be *saying* to him with your punches?"

Johnny yelled out, "I hate you," "You make me sick," and "You're a big jerk" when I instructed him to talk about how he felt. He looked at the bag and stated in a moderately loud voice, "You make me feel mad; you hurt my feelings; you scare me." When he made the last statement I asked some more about feeling afraid. "What's scary about Stevie?" When Johnny could not respond, I told him it was OK, that I wanted him to think about it some more. To conclude I said, "Just like it's not OK for you to hit Stevie, it's not OK for him to hit you. When he hits you, he's doing a bad thing." "He's bad," Johnny punctuated. "When he *hits* you he does a bad thing," I corrected. I wanted to clarify the difference between being inherently bad and doing bad things. Johnny had struggled with self-recriminations about his own hurtful behavior. Then Johnny corrected me, "Larry was bad *and* he did bad things." I did not respond. I asked Johnny to think some more about what was scary about Stevie. My guess was that what scared him the most was the threat of being overwhelmed. His strategy was to be pugnacious as a defense against the threat.

I had met with Johnny for approximately 12 sessions. The first part of the treatment had been purely reactive; we had dealt with the behaviors that were causing the most difficulty to those persons providing his care. Johnny's internal controls were not developed enough to cope with the anxiety, fear, and sense of helplessness originating from his trauma and elicited by normal interactions with peers, caretakers, and his mother. I developed the following treatment plan:

1. Play therapy with Johnny
   a. Set limits on aggressive behavior in and out of treatment.
   b. Continue to discuss good and bad behaviors.
   c. Discuss God and the devil as needed.
   d. Teach appropriate and nondestructive ways to express anger.
   e. Teach Johnny to verbalize feelings of anger.
   f. Discuss and explain children's powers, particularly about choice.
   g. Discuss fears and anxieties and ways of coping.
   h. Discuss sexuality.

2. Parent–child interactions
   a. Help mother set limits with clear and reasonable consequences.
   b. Offer support and direct mother to support services for parents of molested children.
   c. Discuss mother's feelings of guilt about failure to protect Johnny from molestation and her subsequent anger at Johnny's grandmother.
   d. Direct mother away from agitated and nondiscriminatory recounting of the molestation.
   e. Direct mother to provide concrete reassurance to child regarding physical safety (e.g., new locks).
3. Coordination
   a. Make contact with referring party, particularly to discuss what type of information might be necessary to prosecute this case anew.

MIDDLE PHASE OF TREATMENT

As his aggressive behavior seemed to decrease to the normal range for a 5½-year-old boy, Johnny became more verbal regarding sexuality. He had, on occasion, taken a look at my "anatomically correct dolls," exploring the bodies of the male dolls. (He seemed uninterested in the female dolls.) He had usually spent no more than a few seconds in exploration before shoving the dolls away.

At this point in the therapy Johnny turned his attention to the dolls, selecting the small male doll and undressing him completely. He would then take his finger and insert it into the anus of the doll and push inward. He said nothing during this play, avoiding eye contact with me. He would then take down the pants of the adult male doll, being careful to keep them draped around the doll's ankles. He placed the small doll on his stomach and laid the big doll on top. It was weeks before he took the adult doll's penis and put it inside the anus of the small doll. During this time his mother and caretaker reported an escalation of his masturbatory behavior and "dirty talk." I noticed that Johnny became very stiff during this sexual play: He held his breath and appeared dissociative. His play had become fixed at the same instant as he inserted the penis into the small doll's anus.

After I observed this sequence of behavior about ten times, I decided to intervene. The next time he did the sex play I commented, "Larry was wrong to put his penis in your butt." Johnny looked at me extremely surprised. "I want to tell Larry what I think," I continued. "Would that be OK with you?" He acquiesced. "Larry, you were very wrong to put your penis in Johnny's butt. That is a bad thing for a grown-up to do to a child. You made Johnny feel lots of things. Like you made him feel..." I hesitated and leaned over to Johnny, whispering, "What did he make you feel?" "Mad," Johnny mumbled. "Johnny felt mad at you, Larry, because you hurt him and did something bad to him. You also made him feel..." I repeated my cue to Johnny and he again mumbled, "Scared." I talked to Larry in this fashion for quite a while, and Johnny volunteered feelings such as hurt, confused, bad, like crying, like lying, like running, pretending, and "like I couldn't move."

In the subsequent session Johnny took down the pants of the adult male doll and pulled on the doll's penis, attempting to elongate it enough to stick it behind his legs into his own anus. These attempts were not successful, and finally Johnny turned the doll around and inserted a small knife that belonged to one of the toy warriors in the adult doll's anus. "Put that into words," I advised him. Johnny said, "I hate you. I want you to hurt. You feel bad." I affirmed the feeling and not the behavior: "You are mad and want him to feel the same pain you did. Tell him how you feel. Telling him makes you powerful." He yelled insults for a while and seemed satisfied to do so. He threw the Larry doll against the wall, and without prompting he stated, "You were bad to hurt me."

Child Protective Services (CPS) called me because one of Johnny's friends told his mother that Johnny had pulled his pants down in the bathroom. Apparently, Johnny had asked to see his friend's privates, and when the boy refused, Johnny forcibly pulled his pants down. "Johnny," I asked calmly, "did you pull Max's pants down?"

"No," he stated angrily. "Who told you that?"

"Well, Max's mother found out about it, and she called Mrs. Peters because she doesn't want anyone to hurt Max."

"I didn't hurt him," Johnny said. "I could have, but I didn't. I just wanted to see."

"What did you want to see?"

"I wanted to see his privates."

"Why?" I persisted.

"Because...."

"Yes?"

"Because I wanted to."

"Johnny, I want to make a deal with you. When you want to see privates, or talk about privates, or touch privates, I want you to come and talk to me about it. It's not OK to pull kids' pants down, look at their privates, or touch their privates, but we can talk about it together."

"OK," he said unhappily. After obtaining a signed release of information form from his mother, I called the school and told the teacher that I would like her to monitor his play and not allow Johnny to go to the bathroom alone with other children. She informed me that his being alone in the bathroom with another child, which led to the CPS report, had been an isolated incident. Johnny didn't forget my offer to discuss genitals or sexuality. When he first asked to "see" privates, I brought out a set of anatomical drawings (Groth, 1984) and showed him a nude picture of a young male child. I made photocopies of the male child; Johnny asked for a clean copy each week. As he looked at the drawings he laughed, touched the genitalia in the drawing, and used crayons to cover the naked body; afterward, he always crumpled up the drawings and threw them in the garbage. Eventually, Johnny asked if I had a drawing of the adult male. I brought out some photocopies of an anatomical drawing, and he noted that grown-up males have pubic hair. He used a black crayon to cover the midsection of the adult male figure and then made some red spots around the drawing. When I asked him to tell me about the picture, he replied, "Larry cut himself shaving." He smiled and said he was glad Larry was hurt; then he punctured a hole in the drawing. Johnny seemed to be releasing his anger at himself for being unable to stop the abuse and at Larry for abusing him. I usually ended the session by declaring that Larry had been wrong to hurt him and it was not OK to touch or hurt other people's privates.

Johnny was less aggressive in his kindergarten class and in the day-care program after school. He was not, however, an easygoing child; his deportment was oppositional. As his teachers put it, "if you say it's warm, he says it's freezing." This trend was apparent in the therapy sessions. It was critical for Johnny to be correct about everything and have his way all of the time. He claimed to have done everything from skydiving to playing hockey with Prince Charles. His mother found this particularly annoying and frequently accused him of being a liar.

This need to be unconditionally in control seemed to be Johnny's way of managing any feelings of anxiety or helplessness. Although he no longer beat children up or overpowered them physically, he frequently engaged in verbal altercations; as a result, children did not seek him out, and he frequently felt isolated and rejected. These feelings caused him to cultivate a number of defenses including an unyielding stance in which he declared that he liked no one and did not care if anybody liked him or not. Since his social interactions had become so onerous and elicited a consistently disapproving response from others, I decided to put Johnny in a group for little boys with acting-out behavior. He was initially very resistant to attending; by the third session, however, he had developed a camaraderie with the other five boys in the group and seemed to look forward to more meetings.

The group provided Johnny with an opportunity to make contact with other boys his age who had been molested. Johnny announced to me, "Bad things happened to those kids too" when he came to his first individual session following the group meeting. The children were allowed and encouraged to talk about their molestation, asking questions and dealing with specific issues of concern to boy victims, issues like helplessness and homophobia. The children shared generalized fears and anxieties as well as some common problems, such as the struggle to be strong and powerful. In addition, all the children benefited from some exploration of their self-image, self-esteem, aggression, and sexuality. While they had prematurely learned what was *not* all right regarding sexual touching, the group leaders provided information about safe and appropriate touching.

When conflicts arose in the group, they were addressed quickly. The boys soon quickly bonded and the results were immediately visible in individual therapy. For example, Johnny asked quite simply, "How do you get gay?" Apparently, even at his young age, there was some concern that being molested might indicate homosexuality. I referred the question back to the group and consulted with Johnny's mother and the group therapists about a response we could all agree on. The decision was to tell Johnny that no one "becomes" gay because of having been hurt as children; also, children don't get selected to be hurt because of any special reason.

The first year in therapy consisted of addressing themes of aggression, sexuality, social and peer interactions, the victim and perpetrator dyad, helplessness, and empowerment. Johnny had developed a number of defenses to cope with peer rejection that reinforced his feelings of being stigmatized.

An unexpected event altered the course of treatment. Mother had decided to send Johnny to a friend of hers for the holidays. (This friend had a child Johnny's age, and the two children had developed a strong relationship during the school year that was interrupted by the friend's move to a nearby city.) During the visit an unrelated male adult, also spending his holiday with this family, raped Johnny in the middle of the night. The mother called me in despair before picking Johnny up at the airport. Johnny had called her the morning after the abuse and told her what had happened. The family was unaware of the reason for Johnny's sudden decision to return home early, and his mother wanted to see Johnny before telling them more. The rapist had left the house early in the morning.

Johnny was taken directly to the hospital where physical findings were conclusive of sodomy; numerous internal and external injuries confirmed the fact that Johnny had been beaten by the rapist. Immediately following the medical exam, Johnny came to my office. He went into the playroom, grabbed a large stuffed rabbit, and, uncharacteristically, lay on the pillows. He was physically and emotionally fatigued. "I'm so sorry you were hurt," I said. "I can see you want to rest...I'll sit here beside you...If you want to talk, I'll listen." He closed his eyes and seemed almost asleep, and I sat next to him quietly, sharing his pain and fatigue.

The next four months in treatment were unlike any other sessions with Johnny. He was quiet, physically still, and unresponsive. His eyes drooped considerably and he always entered the room and lay down. He was totally shut down. The bruises on his arm had begun to disappear, but his internal scars were quite apparent. Everything gained had been lost. It was a time of despair. Any and all attempts to interact with Johnny were futile. He was uninterested in contact with me, his mother, or the environment. He needed help to stand up, open the door, and find his mother. He was severely depressed and slept a great deal. He lost 10 pounds, which contributed to his frail appearance.

I decided to take Johnny out of the office. We went to the park and although he wouldn't get on the slide or swings, we walked around the park hand in hand. I stopped to get some popcorn for the ducks and noted that Johnny would eat some without prompting. He seemed to enjoy the park, and I asked his mother to try to do some outdoor activities with him, even if he claimed he'd rather stay inside. Mother was unable to get Johnny to go out to the park; since the rape Johnny had been both distant and hostile toward his mother. My interpretation of this was that Johnny felt angry that his mother had failed to protect him from the rape. The twice-weekly outdoor sessions were very successful. Johnny became less physically constricted, eventually running and skipping. He would run ahead of me, more each time; eventually, he played hide-and-seek and did not appear anxious. He climbed trees and reveled in his flourishing physical prowess.

Approximately 4 months after the rape Johnny's mother attended a court hearing, and the rapist was convicted and sent to jail. Johnny proudly proclaimed that "that man has to go to jail. I hope they kill him in jail."

"You're glad the judge sent him to jail," I said.

"Yeah, and now I hope they'll kill him."

"You want him to get hurt the way you were hurt."

"Yeah. I want someone to hurt him."

"He was wrong to hurt you, Johnny."

Johnny seemed to want to stay in the playroom, and the Larry doll was now used interchangeably with the "that man" doll. Johnny would bring the doll down from the shelf, climbing on the sand tray to bring it down himself. He would put the doll behind a chair or hide it under pillows. "He's in jail," he would declare and then throw gorillas, soldiers, dinosaurs, and Ninja Turtles to hurt "that man." "We can't let him out yet," he would whisper. Sometimes he would leave the doll buried from week to week; other times he would return the doll to the shelf before leaving. Often he would ask, "Is Larry in jail too?" I honestly didn't know. Sometimes he would repeat that "Larry was bad" and hurt him when he was "really little." When I asked if he remembered how Larry had hurt him, he said he couldn't remember anymore. He often said that Larry was a "son of Satan" and had "real powers even God can't stop." When Johnny became frightened at night, he would usually verbalize a special fear that Larry might come and "kidnap [him] to a very dark place where no one would ever find [him] again."

DISCUSSION

Johnny was a victim of repeated trauma and suffered from symptoms of posttraumatic stress disorder, including emotionality, nightmares, physical sensations, fear and anxiety, and intrusive flashbacks. These symptoms were manifested by a profusion of behaviors: aggression and sexualized behavior, clinginess and regression, expressed conflict between good and bad (Lucifer and God), and an impaired self-image, including a sense of inherent badness. The first rape had done severe damage, which was exacerbated by a repetition of the same trauma 12 short months later. Johnny's increased sense of well-being and control was greatly diminished by his inability to protect himself from the second rape. His hypervigilance increased and was accompanied by a deep sense of depression and hopelessness.

Fortunately, the therapeutic relationship was well established by the time of the second rape. Johnny was able to come to the therapy sessions and regress without concern for me. This phase of treatment was reparative and focused on Johnny's physical and emotional healing. The first rape had shocked and frightened him; the second one devastated him and generated feelings of futility.

Johnny had periods of time in which he felt and acted helpless. In response, I encouraged autonomy, assigned tasks that could be easily completed, and took Johnny for outdoor sessions, helping him to build physical strength and dexterity by walking, running, climbing.

There were other phases of treatment when Johnny exhibited sexualized and aggressive behaviors toward other children. To assist him in these unrewarding exchanges, which elicited negative and rejecting responses from others, I had his mother bring him to group therapy. In this small, controlled environment his interactions could be carefully monitored, and the interventions from the therapist were consistent and appropriate. The group experience focused on teaching and rewarding positive behaviors and boosting Johnny's identity and self-esteem. Within the group setting the therapists also taught group members about sexuality and types of proper touching between children.

Lastly, the relationship between Johnny and his mother remained afflicted and complicated by the mother's discovery of her own sexual abuse, her ambivalence toward her son, and her guilt for failing to protect him.

The course of treatment included individual therapy, group therapy, family therapy, and two "breaks" from therapy. The first break was during the summer months; the second was related to significant progress in Johnny's social behavior and his now stable enhanced sense of self. There were periodic regressions. Johnny had appendicitis and the sense of helplessness he experienced during his recovery from surgery invoked memories of the rape and his subsequent feelings of physical and emotional fragility. His recovery was slow, fueled by his mother's solicitous behavior. In addition, anniversary dates for the rapes, sometimes consciously acknowledged, summoned dysphoric feelings and/or acting-out behaviors.

Antony: A Child
with Multiple Traumas

REFERRAL INFORMATION

Antony was referred for treatment by his social worker. Antony was physically and sexually abused and neglected; a dependent of the court, Antony lived in a specialized foster home.

SOCIAL/FAMILY HISTORY

Antony, a Hispanic child, was 9 years old at the time of referral. He was one of five children, all of whom had different fathers. The three younger siblings had been released for adoption; Antony and his 15-year-old sister, Sarah, were in separate long-term foster homes.

Antony's parents, Jose and Lupe, had a fleeting relationship that ended abruptly when Jose was shot during a drug transaction. Lupe had numerous brief encounters; her children never had contact with their respective fathers.

Lupe had been drug-dependent since she was a teenager. She was sexually abused by her father and expelled from her family when she disclosed this fact; she had been called a slut by her mother and older sisters and told never to return to the house. She told the social worker that she had then stayed with some girlfriends off and on and eventually met a man who took her in, fed her, bought her clothes, and seemed to ask little in return. Unfortunately, the man turned out to be a pimp, and Lupe was introduced into the "working life" on the streets of Los Angeles. Lupe claims that her first encounter with marijuana was with a "trick" who offered her a quick high. She found that being stoned allowed her to go numb, a sensation she very much enjoyed. Since that time she had smoked marijuana daily and in the last 2 years had become a multiple-drug user, trading sex for drugs.

In spite of the drug dependency and prostitution, Lupe was able to provide sporadic marginal care for her two older children. She had occasionally been able to pay rent and live with her children, and some of her friends had offered them temporary respite. She had always wanted children and held firm to her assertion that she loved them all very much; releasing her small children for adoption was viewed by Lupe as her most noble gift to them. She had a tubal ligation following the birth of her last child, who was born with massive brain damage due to Lupe's drug use.

Lupe has entered drug treatment programs cyclically. She is currently in a state-funded residential drug rehabilitation program, and her prognosis is guarded. She has had less than three visits with each of her elder children in the last 2 years. Sarah has been in the same foster home for the last 4 years, and she has made a good adjustment to her foster parents, who have expressed an interest in adopting her. Lupe has been reluctant to release this child, her firstborn, for adoption.

Antony's experience in foster homes has been unstable: He has been in approximately eight different foster homes. He was also considered for adoption at one time, yet Lupe was reluctant to release him for adoption as well; no steps were taken to terminate parental rights. Antony has had a range of troublesome behaviors n foster care; some of his transfers were precipitated by requests from the foster parents.

When treatment began, Antony had been transferred to a "specialized" foster home after stealing some money in his foster home. The social work department viewed the child's stealing as a "child failing placement," and requested therapy for Antony's "acting-out behavior."

CLINICAL IMPRESSIONS

Antony was a small, shy boy with constricted movement and flattened affect. He said little, moved slowly, and seemed resistant to being in my office; his foster mother stated that he had locked himself in his room, refusing to come to the session. Antony had acquiesced to come out of his room and come to therapy because she offered him a dollar's worth of quarters for the video machine near the house.

I had met with the foster mother, Mrs. R., prior to the appointment with Antony. She described Antony as a quiet, shy child who seemed to be "totally shut down." She reported no problems at the time of our meeting, adding that the social worker had cautioned her that Antony is always at his best when he first arrives at a new foster home. Mrs. R. stated that Antony would not eat during mealtime but raided the refrigerator constantly. His sleeping pattern seemed erratic; often, she would awaken at night to find him listening to his radio or reading some comic books he had brought with him. He seemed to have a particular penchant for superheroes, not uncommon for children his age.

The most difficult problem she noted was Antony's hygiene: He played hard, sweating profusely, and refused to take showers. In the 2 weeks he had been with her, he had taken one shower and then only when he was offered a reward. He took his dirty clothes out of the clothes hamper and wanted to wear the same clothes 3 or 4 days in a row. Mrs. R. had not forced him to change and had asked for suggestions regarding this behavior. I told her that she was doing the right thing by not insisting that Antony bathe or change and that I would give her some advice as soon as I met with him and got to know him a little.

Mrs. R. had been a specialized foster parent for 4 years, and her home was licensed for four children who required special attention. When Antony was placed with her, there were two smaller girls in the home. Antony had reportedly displayed some aggression toward boys in other settings but seemed protective of girls.

THE BEGINNING PHASE OF TREATMENT

Antony did not display any acting-out behavior initially. The social worker had reiterated her observation to me that Antony always made a very good first impression and developed difficult behavior later on.

At first, Antony was quiet and lethargic; he entered the playroom displaying little interest or enthusiasm. He asked nothing and picked out a book to read; he read continuously for most of the session, hardly interacting with me. He spoke few words, did not make eye contact with me, and did not ask to play with any of the toys within reach or on the top shelves. My only comment to him was, "I am someone kids can talk with and share their thoughts and feelings with." I added, "Lots of kids don't like coming here at first." I had explained that the bell on the timer would ring when it was time for him to leave. He seemed oblivious when the bell rang, apparently impartial about leaving or staying.

I decided to be nondirective with Antony. He had experienced numerous placements and had encountered an assortment of new environments and caretakers. According to the social worker, he had been interviewed myriad times by police and by personnel of the child protective services agency. Some of his foster parents had remarked with disdain that Antony "never gave anything back, except trouble." He had been labeled "uncooperative, capricious, and selfish." Apparently, his caretakers had expected a reciprocal relationship, and Antony was not motivated to socialize.

My nondirective approach was respectful of Antony's attachment disorder. I did not expect him to trust me or be interested in yet another short-lived relationship. My job was to become trustworthy and to become consistent in his life.

Weekly appointments were unremarkable for the first 3 months. Antony would bring books to read to himself, play quietly with small cars that crashed into each other, listen to music on a Walkman, and generally ignore me. I sat nearby on the floor and engaged in parallel play. Sometimes I read or colored or took small cars off the shelf to examine. I noted the position of power he retained throughout the sessions. I could understand how caretakers had difficulty with his apathetic yet provocative behavior.

During the fourth month of treatment, Mrs. R. was hospitalized for emergency surgery, and her sister moved in as temporary caretaker. This event engendered the first shift in the therapy. Antony came into the playroom with a sense of urgency; he sat on the big pillows and crossed his arms in front of him. "I hate her," he announced. "You hate who?" I inquired. "Rosa—she thinks she's in charge of me, but she's not. Nobody's in charge of me. Fuck that bitch." I had never heard Antony speak so much, and with so much affect. I was very pleased.

"You don't like Rosa telling you what to do."

"Hell no. And if she doesn't chill out, I'm going to show her what's what."

"What are you feeling right now, Antony?"

"I'm pissed."

"What are you pissed about?"

"Rosa. She thinks she can make me do stuff."

"What did she say or do that made you feel pissed?"

"She says I got to wear a clean shirt to school. I don't like doing that. I feel like a wimp when I'm all clean."

"What do you usually do when Mrs. R. is home?"

"She lets me decide."

"Maybe Rosa doesn't know."

"She won't listen to me. She thinks she's so smart."

I took a big risk. "Antony, let me have Rosa come in here for just a few minutes, and let's see if we can get this worked out."

"Hell no. I'm outahere if she comes."

"Antony. You don't have to do or say anything. Just let me see if I can help her understand."

"She won't."

"OK. Let me try."

I walked out of the playroom and spoke to Rosa, telling her that I understood how difficult it must be to be worried about her sister and to take care of these children who missed her. She teared up and said she thought she was in over her head. I offered to meet with her the next day if she could arrange child care for the younger children. I asked if she was aware that Antony was angry; she was not. He had been very sullen about something, but she wasn't sure why. When I explained about the shirt, she remembered the incident in the morning but was unaware of the significance the incident held for him. I was eager to facilitate a positive exchange between Rosa and Antony.

We all sat down and I said, "Antony is angry because he wants to decide what to wear to school." Rosa spontaneously said, "Antony, I'm sorry, I didn't know you could decide...the shirt looked a little dirty to me. I didn't want you to be embarrassed at school." Antony sat, arms crossed, silent. "Antony is really good at listening and paying attention. He doesn't always use words to express himself," I told her.

"I know how that can be," Rosa added. "I get shy myself with people I don't know."

I took the opportunity to say to Rosa, "It must be so hard for all of you that Mrs. R. is in the hospital. You must be worried." "She's going to be fine," Rosa responded, "It was just so sudden." "I don't like surprises myself," I said, "and for the children it must be twice as hard, because they've had lots of surprises in their lives."

Rosa left and Antony blurted, "She was nice 'cause you were here."

"Well, I'm glad you don't have to be angry about your school clothes anymore."

"I wouldn't have put them on anyway."

"Anything else you might be angry about, Antony?"

"No."

He took down the cars and crashed them into the walls.

By the time he left his body was less tense. Surprisingly he said, "See you next week."

From that session on there was verbal dialogue—nevertheless. Mrs. R. was out of the home for 3 weeks, and when she returned a live-in nurse provided assistance. When Mrs. R. came home, she brought the children little presents. Antony brought in his present: a game of Chinese checkers. It was brand-new and, apparently, the first brand-new toy he had ever had: He delighted in telling me that it had come with a plastic wrapper and that he had torn it off himself. He played intensely, concentrating on every move. He was proud when he won and eager to play again when he lost. His losses were infrequent.

Although there had been a shift in the therapy when Antony was able to talk to me about his anger, he continued to constrict the expression of his feelings. I used a set of cards that had illustrations of faces demonstrating a wide range of feelings. I thought that Antony might be able to select the cards depicting feelings like those he had about people or situations, and I was impressed by his ability to use the cards in a variety of ways. I brought in the cards in their wrapper and told Antony I had just gotten something new in the mail. He was intrigued and opened the box. At first, we played by picking a card and telling each other about a time we remembered having the feeling depicted on the card. Later, I would ask Antony to communicate using the cards. For example, I inquired, "When Mrs. R. went to the hospital, how did you feel?" He picked three cards: "Mad," "Sad," and "Disappointed."

"I remember how angry you were when you came to see me the week Mrs. R. went to the hospital. You remember that?"

"Yeah."

"You were mad because Rosa made you wear your clean shirt that day."

"That's right."

"What else do you think you were angry about?"

"My foster mom going to the hospital." It was the first time he'd ever called her mom. He had become attached to

Mrs. R., perhaps responding to her gentle, nonintrusive approach.

"I understand being mad about that, Antony." He reached his tolerance level and brought out the Chinese checkers.

Treatment Plan

1. Be consistent; become trustworthy. Avoid cancellations or rescheduling.
2. Be nondirective: Give Antony a sense of freedom; don't intrude.
3. Assess for underlying depression.
4. Document play themes and sequence of play.
5. Introduce nonintrusive interactions, parallel play.
6. Assist in the expression of feelings.
7. Long-term goals: discuss feelings about biological family; father's shooting; siblings' adoption.
8. Meet monthly with Mrs. R. or as necessary.
9. Stay in touch with social worker regarding the foster placement, mother's treatment progress, and any reunification plans.

THE MIDDLE PHASE OF TREATMENT

The "feeling cards" remained an effectual means of communication between Antony and me, and other techniques became useful as well. Antony discovered the puppets and storytelling: He would crawl behind something, hold his puppets high above himself, and tell stories rich with symbolism. One of his favorite stories follows:

RABBIT: Welcome to my land of surprises. Many things happen in this world. But I can't say more. Someone's coming. I've got to go.

SPIDER: Well, I've got some surprises in store. I'm a tarantula, and I have strong poison, and I come up behind someone and attack quickly. Death is quick. No one knows what causes death. I surprise them all with death. I have much deadly power. I run fast, and no one knows how to catch me. Just watch.

TEDDY BEAR: Ho hum, what a nice day. The sun is out; the sky is blue. Honey's in the tree. Yum, yum. OUCH! WHAT WAS THAT??? THAT HURTS. (*He falls down dead.*)

SQUIRREL: Ho hum, what a nice day. The sun is out, the sky is blue. Nuts are in the tree. Yum, yum. OUCH! WHAT WAS THAT??? THAT HURTS. (*He falls down dead.*)

RABBIT: You have to be really careful around here. Even though you can't see it, there are dangers all around. I've had to take great precautions. See my muscles. I've had to pump myself up. I stay away, 'cause I always know just when to take off. And now's the time.

There are several themes of relevance in this story. There is a perceived but camouflaged danger. The danger, symbolized by the spider, is lethal and attacks quickly. The spider enjoys the power of killing and seems to select vulnerable targets (symbolized by a squirrel and a teddy bear).

Although Antony's stories always reflected a dangerous environment and potential death, in the middle phase of therapy he developed the rabbit character, who always told the story and always managed to escape. The rabbit was always hypervigilant, always resourceful, and intent on developing physical strength. This was a good prognostic sign and marked Antony's switch from learned helplessness to an increased sense of empowerment. Also, the stories reflected optimism, not futility.

Throughout the middle phase of treatment the rabbit continued to appear in sundry stories, and he encountered earthquakes, floods, and other catastrophes. He always escaped, sometimes just in the nick of time. His physical strength enabled him to leap great distances, fight numerous adversaries, and climb steep mountains. Concurrently, Antony was on a soccer team with a winning record, and he was exhilarated by his indisputable skills in kicking, running, and manipulating the ball. His self-esteem and confidence were greatly enhanced by the fact that his teammates heralded him for his propensity for making goals, and Antony greatly enjoyed winning. Moreover, Mrs. R. attended every game, a fact that did not go unnoticed by Antony.

Antony continued to avoid verbalizing his feelings. At the same time, he was most receptive to communicating through other means. I would often draw a figure of a man or woman with a circle above them, as cartoonists do with their characters' dialogue. "Who is this?" I would ask Antony, and he would volunteer names, such as those of his foster mother, his teacher, or a girl he liked. He would sometimes direct me to draw a new figure of a "kid in a karate suit," and he would then speak through this character. One day I drew a woman with a smaller figure at her side. "This is you, and this is your mom," I said. I sat back and commented, "I wonder what you would say to your mom and she would say to you." He filled in the cartoon mother's circle with: "You sure are strong." He left his blank. The topic of his mother was tremendously onerous for Antony.

During one memorable session, I told a story about a mother squirrel and her baby squirrel. The story consisted of a mother squirrel who very much loved her baby and yet was always leaving him behind, citing work responsibilities and urgent appointments that had to be kept. The little squirrel was very confused. How could a mother who loved her baby leave him alone? "No way," Antony said, "she's full of excuses." Antony had both a fear of discussing his mother and a wish to do so. The symbolism allowed the distance he wanted and needed. "I don't want to talk about this anymore," he said. He abruptly began kicking the punching bag. My opening was made.

The next session I had placed the baby squirrel under a pillow. "Look," I told Antony, "the baby's feeling really down. He misses his mom so much." "I know," he said, "let's make her come back." "OK," I agreed. (I would follow his lead on this theme, no matter where he wanted to go.) He got the mother squirrel and brought her out. "OK, OK, quit your balling," said Antony in a high pitched voice as he took the mother to the pillow. "You need to take care of yourself; I won't always be around." I jumped in and asked Antony what the baby should say. He whispered what I should make the baby say, and I relayed his message: "Mom, I'm too little to be by myself." The mother was harsh as she said, "No you're not. You're a boy. You've got to be tough. If you're not tough, other guys will hurt you and make mince pie out of you." I asked him how the baby would respond and he didn't know. I whimpered and had the baby squirrel say, "Mommy, please don't leave me. I want you to be with me." Antony threw the mother squirrel into the wall, and the role play abruptly ended. I waited. Antony went to the corner and sat there, holding his face in his hands. He seemed to be crying, and I didn't want to do or say anything to deter his first show of appropriate sadness at the loss of his mother. Finally, he said, "Why can't my mom take care of me?"

"Why do you think?" I asked softly.

"She can't stop taking drugs."

"That's right," I said, "and because she's on drugs she can barely take care of herself, let alone take care of you."

"Shit...why is she so stupid?"

"It's OK to be angry at her, Antony. You want her to be a mom to you."

"She's so stupid," he went on. "She meets these dopeheads and brings them home. They pay her to have sex with her. It's gross." I had always suspected that Antony had witnessed his mother's prostitution; he had been overheard making explicit sexual comments to other children. "You worry she might get hurt, huh?"

"Once," Antony gained momentum, "a guy was beating her up, and I took a bottle and broke it over his head. Then my mom and I got away."

"You've taken care of her sometimes, Antony."

"Can we go out?" he asked.

"Sure," I responded. "I know it's hard to talk about your mom...you have so many different feelings about her."

After this session talking about his mother was easier for Antony. When he wanted to say or ask something or ask about her, he would grab the small squirrel. "Do you think she thinks about me?" he asked sincerely.

"I'm sure she does."

"Will I ever live with her again?" he asked another time.

"I honestly don't know," I told him. "It depends on whether she can get off the drugs and learn to take care of herself."

And still another time he asked, "How old do you think I'll be when I get to live with her?" I was sorry to give him yet another "I don't know" answer.

Since Antony had opened the door, I approached him with an idea early in one of our sessions: "What would you think about writing a letter to your mom?" He seemed defensive as he asked what I meant. I explained that it would be possible for us to work on writing a letter together, and he could then decide if he wanted to mail it to her. I had recently contacted the social worker, and I was aware that Antony's mother was reportedly making progress in the rehabilitation program she had entered after a detoxification program. The social worker had been quick to caution that his mother usually made progress early in the treatment. We had discussed the fact that if the progress continued, we might arrange a phone or face-to-face contact between Antony and his mother, supervised by me.

The possibility of Antony having contact with his mother seemed somewhat realistic. Antony had made great strides himself. He was more communicative, expressing some of his feelings. He had made a good attachment to his foster mother, and he was involved in a soccer team at school. His aggressive behaviors were on the decline, and he had improved his personal hygiene. Most important, he relied on the therapy and used it to his benefit, frequently bringing in questions and concerns. He would always tell me about altercations with friends and/or teachers at school; likewise, he would bring in school papers and report cards, proudly showing areas of improvement. Antony was responding well to the continuity provided by his foster placement, his therapy, his karate lessons, and other activities promoted by his foster mother, such as Sunday school. He had made a friend, he had lost 8 pounds, and he bathed every other day. In addition, Mrs. R.'s dog had puppies, and one of them had been given to Antony as a reward for his cooperative spirit and his helpful attitude around the house. It was clear that a special bond had developed between Mrs. R. and Antony, perhaps inspired by their shared cultural background.

I wondered if Antony's progress would be impeded if there were contact between Antony and his mother; his sense of well-being was newly found and fragile. Although positive changes had occurred, sustaining them over time was uncertain. If Antony could use his new skills and apply his new confidence to challenges, disappointments, and difficulties in the future, he would be fortified by his strengths rather than devastated by life's difficulties.

Antony thought long and hard before deciding to write a letter to his mother, and he approached the piece of paper with visible trepidation. Several times he simply stated, "I got nothing to say." I encouraged him by saying, "I'm sure something will come to you." His first letter was painfully brief, and yet he seemed anxious to try again. The first letter read as follows:

"Dear mom. How are you? It's been a long time. Maybe you can write. Antony."

The second letter:

"Dear mom. How are you? I think about you. I hope you are eating good foods."

And the third:

"Dear mom. I think about you sometimes. How are you doing?"

Antony did not persevere. He was uninterested in contact with his mother. His mother, however, encouraged by her drug counselor, decided to write a letter to Antony. He brought the letter to me 3 weeks after receipt. "My mom sent me this letter."

"Oh," I responded. "What does she say?"

"I didn't read it yet."

"I see," I responded, again proceeding with extreme caution. "Do you think you might read it sometime?"

Antony responded without hesitation, "I want you to read it."

I remarked, "You want me to read it to you." He turned away from me and mumbled a positive response. I opened the letter and read aloud:

Dear Tony:

It seems so strange to be writing you. I close my eyes and think of you as you were when I last saw you. I am happy to hear that you are doing well in your foster home. I have called and talked to the social worker and she says you and Sarita are doing good. That is what I want for both of you. I am just learning about me and how to stop making the mistakes I have in the past. One thing I want you to know is that I never stop loving you and hoping your life can be better. I do want to keep getting clean and sober. After that, I hope maybe we can talk, or meet to say hello. I know I have a long way to go and I hope when you think of me you have forgiveness in your heart. I find that praying to our God helps me forgive. I hope you will turn to God too. If you can, send me a picture of you. I want to see how big you are now.

Your mother

I folded the letter and held it, waiting for Antony to say something or turn around. I heard a sniffle, and he touched his face. He was holding some little cars and handed me one asking for a race. We played with the cars for a while, and I waited for him to say something. He did not.

The session passed slowly. Antony was obviously affected by the words he heard, but he would not comment. When the bell rang, I handed him the letter saying, "Thanks for bringing it here and letting me read it to you, Antony. Maybe next week you can tell me how you felt hearing from your mom."

The next session he brought a letter he had written to his mom and a school picture he wanted to include. His letter was brief and moving:

Dear Mami:

Thanks for writing me. I think of you sometimes too and I am happy you are not using drugs now. If you learns how to stay away from the drugs—at school they teach us to Just Say No—maybe someday we can see each other.

I play soccer very good now and in the picture I have my uniform on. I do pray some nights.

Tony

He wanted me to correct his spelling; and there were just a few minor errors. He copied the letter to a new piece of paper, and we called the social worker to get his mother's address. We walked to the corner, and when Antony put the letter in the mailbox, he looked happy.

The following week Antony greeted me and stated, "She hasn't written me again."

I said, "How will you feel if she does?"

Antony responded, "Like it, I guess."

"And how will you feel if she doesn't?"

Antony shrugged his shoulders. "She probably won't."

"And if she doesn't, how will you feel?"

"I don't care," he said quickly.

I took his hand to get his attention and stated, "Antony, it's OK to want something to happen. If it doesn't, you might feel disappointed, angry, or sad. That would be normal. You've been disappointed by your mom a lot."

He didn't pull away and said, "Yeah." Then he asked, "Do you think she'll get off the drugs?"

I answered honestly: "It's a very hard thing to do, and your mom has been on drugs a very long time. We can all hope for the best, and pray for her, but I don't know if the treatment will work or not."

"I know. She's been in lots of programs before."

Antony was in treatment for another 8 months following the sessions just described. He began wanting to do other things after school and asked me if he could go to soccer practice or football practice instead of coming to see me. I told him that it was all right with me, since so many things had changed for him and he was no longer having the kind of problems he had before.

I asked him if he thought anything could happen that would make him feel bad or angry or sad and make him feel like coming to see me again. He said, "If I had to go live with someone else" and added, "If I had to go live with my mom again." His mother had not made contact again, and Antony seemed to reconcile himself to not expecting anything from her in order to avoid the disappointment that could follow. As soon as he told me these things he looked up and said, "I can come back if I have to, right?" It was as if he wanted to make sure I wasn't going anywhere. "Of course," I responded. "You have my number and can call me anytime."

We had four termination sessions, in which we reviewed Antony's drawings and talked about all the different things we had discussed and the different ways we had communicated feelings. We also talked about his resources in the future and who he felt he could turn to if he needed help of any kind. He named Mrs. R., his soccer coach, and his friend Pablo from the team. Antony had clearly formed some positive attachments. Mrs. R. was a long-term placement, and chances were that Antony would continue in her care until majority unless something unforeseen occurred.

DISCUSSION

Antony was a victim of physical and sexual abuse and neglect. The specifics of his abuse never surfaced during therapy. He was referred because of his alternately depressed and aggressive behaviors. This child had suffered great instability during his formative years and had experienced few positive attachments or consistency. He seemed unmotivated to socialize with others, and his poor hygiene might have been a way to isolate himself from others.

During the course of treatment numerous significant events occurred. Antony formed a strong affinity for Mrs. R., his foster mother, and she was tender and affectionate with him. She signed Antony up for the soccer team at school and took him to Sunday school at her church. Antony thrived physically in soccer and enjoyed being part of a team. He also showed a quiet interest in Catholicism.

In treatment, Antony learned to identify his feelings and express them. Although he could not express them verbally at first, eventually he learned to communicate in a more direct way. Antony's relationship to his mother remained conflicted. He had extremely ambivalent feelings toward her; he both wanted her and wanted to reject her. His best defense was to appear indifferent to her in an effort to escape unhurt. He responded to her overture to him but remained uncertain about approaching her. As is typical of neglected children, Antony responded well to appropriate and positive interactions with others.

Gabby: A Child Traumatized by a Single Episode of Sexual Abuse

REFERRAL INFORMATION

Gabby, a 3½-year-old girl, was referred to treatment by her mother after she was orally copulated and digitally penetrated by two adolescent boys, who had occasionally babysat for the child. Her mother had been referred by the pediatrician who treated the child for genital trauma.

SOCIAL/FAMILY HISTORY

Gabby was the second child of divorced parents, Denise and Gustavo. She had an older sibling, Matthew, age 12. Denise and Gustavo were divorced soon after Gabby's birth, after years of a "difficult and strained" relationship. There had been a custody dispute and joint custody was awarded. Gustavo had accused Denise of being "cold and distant" with him and the children and spending more time and energy on her career than on taking care of the home. Denise had accused Gustavo of being practically a "stranger" to his own children. She claimed the only reason he was disputing her sole custody of the children was because he thought that meant he would have to pay more in child support. The parents had unresolved issues between them, reflected in their curt and tense communication. I asked Denise to notify Gustavo about her request to have Gabby in therapy with me and about my desire to meet with both of them individually to get their important perceptions about Gabby. Gustavo had been unconvinced that therapy was necessary but deferred to the pediatrician, whose opinion he valued.

Gustavo was the oldest sibling of his family and had three younger sisters. He described his childhood as happy and referred to his mother with great reverence, citing her sacrificial commitment to the family. His father was depicted as a stern disciplinarian and a scholar. His mother maintained a close relationship with Gustavo and, he reported, would give her eyeteeth to raise Gabby "properly."

Denise was the only child in her family. Her mother was the first in her family to obtain a college degree and to get a divorce. Denise quickly added that her mother balanced home and career extremely well and that she felt the divorce had little impact on her. She stated that her relationship with her father had been positive and that she had always been able to count on him even though he lived on the East Coast and she and her mother had moved to the West Coast after the divorce. Denise added that her mother had been a wonderful and available grandmother, who was able to keep her opinions to herself and let Denise make the parental decisions regarding Gabby.

Denise and Gustavo had met in college and been good friends prior to becoming romantic. Denise described their marriage as "never having a chance," due to her mother-in-law's meddling. She stated that Gustavo always compared her to his mother and that she never rose to his expectations of what a good wife should be.

Gustavo claimed that he would have been willing to work on the marriage but felt that Denise's feminist ideas would not permit her to be a "decent" mother and a scientist at the same time.

Denise worked in a university-based cancer research program, and Gustavo worked as an architect with the City Planning Commission.

Both parents spoke positively about both children. They exulted in their son's academic achievements and his abundant awards in gymnastics. They both agreed that the children had a warm and easygoing relationship with each other, with occasional "normal" manifestations of sibling rivalry. In particular, when Gustavo took Matthew for hiking or fishing outings, Gabby sulked for hours because her Papi had left her behind.

Both parents also acknowledged the sadness and fears expressed by both children when they were told of the divorce. Gustavo noted that the children had complained to him that they missed him and wished he would come home soon.

The sexual abuse of Gabby took place when the parents' usual babysitter, a girl of 13 who lived nearby, entertained her boyfriend and his two friends in Gabby's home. While the children slept and the babysitter and her boyfriend were necking in the living room, the other two boys found and entered Gabby's bedroom, apparently fondling her in her sleep. The sexual molestation escalated; one of the boys performed oral sex while the other one masturbated himself and inserted his fingers in the little girl's vagina. Some bruising around Gabby's mouth suggested that one of the boys had covered her mouth during the abuse. The boys later told police that they scared the little girl and told her if she told anybody what they did, they would kill her.

When Denise came home from a late meeting, she paid the babysitter and went to sleep. When Gabby came into her bedroom in the morning, she knew immediately something was wrong. The child had blood around her legs and black-and-blue marks around her mouth. Mother rushed the child to the pediatrician, who filed a report with Child Protective Services. Mother gave the police the babysitter's name, and a meeting with her uncovered the boys' presence at the house.

The boys went to juvenile court, were placed on probation, and were referred for treatment.

During my intake meetings with both Denise and Gustavo, they concurred that Gabby was anxious, fearful, and insomniac, waking frequently with nightmares. She wanted to sleep with her mother, and Denise had acquiesced in order to make her feel safe enough to sleep through the night. Gabby had shied away from her brother and father, apparently reluctant to have physical contact with them. (She did sleep through the night at her father's house, usually fretfully.) Her parents also reported that Gabby was lethargic and was exhibiting regressed behavior such as thumbsucking and baby talk. In addition, she was no longer able or willing to use the toilet by herself and insisted that her mother and/or her day-care worker take her to the toilet and keep diapers on her. Both parents expressed concern for Matthew, who was feeling guilty that he had not awakened when his sister was in trouble and who was furious at the boys who had hurt her. I referred him to a colleague for an assessment and brief therapy.

CLINICAL IMPRESSIONS

My first meeting with Gabby was brief. She would not separate from her mother and dug her face into her mother's lap, unwilling to speak to me or come look at the playroom. I assured Denise that this was to be expected and told her that I wanted her to take the child into the playroom without me and show her around. Denise told me that Gabby had looked around with moderate attention but had resisted touching anything and wanted to leave soon after they entered the room.

At the second meeting Gabby continued to avoid eye contact with me. There were some other children her age in the waiting room, playing with building blocks, and Gabby appeared somewhat interested. I sat in the waiting room with her, encouraging her interest and participation in play with the others. Eventually, Gabby approached and stood next to them but ran back to her mother when the children greeted her.

I invited Denise and Gabby into the playroom, and Gabby seemed to look around as I told her about the different things in the room. I introduced myself in typical fashion, that is, as someone who talks to children about their thoughts and feelings. I explained she could choose the toys she wanted to play with, and I reviewed the use of the timer. I talked to her mother so that Gabby would feel safer, telling her that some children like to color in the coloring books, some children like to play with the cups and saucers, and so forth.

Gabby looked upward when I told her that all the children who came to see me had been hurt by somebody. "Some of the kids have hurts on their bodies; some of them have hurt feelings." She actually gave a little smile when I mentioned that the children don't ever have to talk about their hurts, that sometimes they just play. Gabby sucked her thumb as I colored in the book with her mother, the two of us conversing about her early history. Gabby listened quietly as her mother described her as a baby and told about the kinds of things she had liked to do. Denise said that one of Gabby's favorite things was the beach and swimming. They had taken a vacation to Hawaii not too long ago, and Gabby, with a mask on her face, had loved peering into the water and watching the fish. I told Gabby that I had also been in Hawaii and loved the fish and the beaches and the hula dancers. (She smiled again.)

In the third session I brought out my sand tray, and Gabby became consumed with interest in the sand play—so much so that I told Gabby her mother would be waiting outside the playroom today, that I would place a chair for her right outside the door and leave the door open. At one point Gabby looked up and seemed to panic as she asked for her mother. "She's right outside the door. Go look," I said; Gabby ran to make sure her mother was there. She then returned on her own and continued her play in the sand.

The initial sessions consisted of Gabby's filling up cups and emptying them, and wetting the sand and building little hills she would then poke holes in. She loved smoothing out the sand and bunching it up. She had noticed the shelves full of little miniatures that stood next to the sand tray. She had picked some of the miniatures up, quickly returning them to their exact location.

Her mother's chair was still next to the door by the fifth session, but the door remained closed. Gabby separated quietly, apparently no longer disturbed by the separation, more confident that her mother would wait for her to finish her session. Eventually, I moved the chair back to the waiting room; after checking once to see that her mother was still there, Gabby never required her mother's presence in or near the playroom again.

Treatment Planning

I developed the following treatment plan:

1. Individual play therapy
   a. Allow nondirective, nonintrusive play.
   b. Document play themes and interpret symbolism.
   c. Facilitate posttraumatic play.
   d. Facilitate Gabby's sharing of dreams.
2. Parent-child sessions
   a. Meet with parents and discuss Gabby's behaviors and suggested responses.
   b. Discourage overprotective responses.
   c. Discuss sleeping arrangements.
3. Sibling
   a. Meet with siblings together; Matt might want to share his feelings with sister, if appropriate.
   b. Encourage renewed physical contact through specific games.
4. Family
   a. Family meeting to symbolize the abuse being in the past and to discuss ways that Gabby will be safe in the future.

THE BEGINNING PHASE OF TREATMENT

Gabby had endured a terrifying traumatic event, the terror intensified by the fact that the event had occurred in the safety of her home. When the trauma is external to the home, the child seeks, and hopefully obtains, reassurance from her immediate environment; when the trauma occurs in the immediate environment, reassurance is less possible.

Because of Gabby's young age, I postulated that the sexual abuse had not been perceived necessarily as a sexual event but, rather, as an act of violence and physical intrusion. It was also likely that she had been terrorized by having her mouth and nose covered, and may even have lost consciousness (as the boys who abused her had "guessed").

The child had regressed developmentally: She was clingy, wanted diapers, and resorted to single words to signal what she wanted rather than the full sentences she had used prior to the trauma. She exhibited symptoms of post-traumatic stress, including night terrors, intrusive flash-backs, emotionality, dissociative episodes, and feelings of numbing. Gabby also had specific trepidation associated with males, both within and outside her family. Both her mother and father had observed that Gabby could not tolerate talking with men or being around them. (Denise said Gabby would not look at men and started to cry; Gustavo stated that when a male appeared, she became insistent on leaving the surroundings straightaway.)

My immediate goals were to create a safe environment and to facilitate Gabby's processing of the traumatic event. I kept verbal communication to a minimum and allowed the child to choose her preferred play materials. I had gently introduced her to the playroom, allowing her mother to reassure and comfort her as needed. Slowly, Gabby began to tolerate being alone with me in the playroom. I told her she could say as much or as little as she wanted, choose what to play with, enter or exit the room as needed, and stay until the timer went off. She had permission to check on her mother outside the playroom, and did so sporadically for the first few months in therapy.

Although initially Gabby colored, used the cups and saucers in the sand, and even combed the hair on some of the dolls, eventually the sand tray became the nucleus of her attention as she began her difficult journey into recovery. The sand tray was always smoothed down first. Then Gabby would begin the slow and purposeful process of selecting small miniatures for her tray, placing them carefully on a platform that slid out from under the tray. She took painstaking care to dip each little figure in a cup of water, eliminating the grains of sand that had become attached during play. She always organized the figures, making a line of dinosaurs, lions and tigers, spiders and bugs, and soldiers with swords and guns. Then she picked out green, yellow, and white fences. The green fences were the tallest; the white and yellow ones served as reinforcers and were placed in front of the green. The last level collected were the trees, and Gabby picked both tall and shorter ones, placing them in front of the fence.

Gabby's play was identical each week for the first 3 months of therapy: She would smooth out the sand, clean and dry each figure, set them out in lines, and begin to fill in the sand tray. First, she would put a small figure, Garfield the cat, in the left hand corner of the tray. She covered it midway with sand and then proceeded to place the tallest fence about 3 inches in front of the Garfield figure. She would reinforce the fence, and then place the trees in front of the fences. Then, starting from the farthest end of the tray, she would fill in the remaining three-quarters of the tray with (threatening) figures, including dinosaurs, spiders and bugs, lions and tigers, and soldiers, the latter being closest to the fence (see Figure 1). Spontaneously, Gabby noted, "They climb trees and jump fences." The implication was clear: The boundaries were permeable and attack was inevitable. The single object in the corner could not hide, and no one was around to come to his aid.

At the beginning this was a stable, undynamic tray; the figures would not move. Gabby seemed to have an internal clock so that she would finish setting up the tray just when it was time for her session to end. Gabby was absorbed by the play, seemingly unaware of my presence or outside noises. She would become visibly anxious as she placed all the threatening objects in the tray. She could not tolerate looking at them for too long, and sometimes she mumbled "Oh, oh," as if something bad were going to happen.

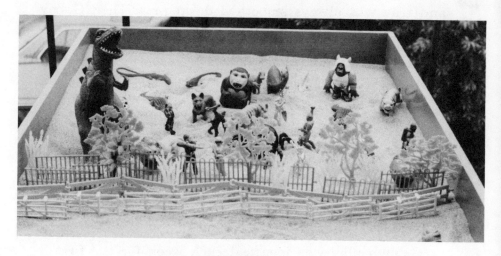

FIGURE 1

THE MIDDLE PHASE OF TREATMENT

A shift in Gabby's sand play scenario began to take place ever
so subtly. The fence was retreating from the Garfield object,
the space with the threatening objects was contracting, and
fewer threatening objects were invading.

By the end of the fourth month half the tray was filled
with soldiers and a few random animals; Garfield was now
joined by a giraffe, towering over the fences, and a bear,
looking confident and unperturbed by all the danger. When
she worked on the tray during this phase of her treatment,
Gabby would sometimes turn her attention to another toy
before the bell rang; she was leaving herself some time to do
something akin to reorienting to the environment. And she
always waved good-bye to the tray and to me as she left.

Gabby's behavior had progressed tremendously at home.

She was sleeping through the night more frequently, with only occasional nightmares. She had responded well to an intervention of finger painting with her brother, sharing the same piece of paper. This gave the siblings an opportunity to have nonthreatening physical contact while having a positive experience together. They had also shared the task of kneading dough for a pizza, laughing and having fun while they had close contact with each other. Gustavo had even joined in the finger painting once, and although Gabby had liked it, she had wondered why her dad was acting so silly.

Denise reported that Gabby's crying bouts had decreased, as had those periods in which she seemed to "stare out into the wilderness." Gustavo acknowledged the recovery that had occurred and felt it was time to terminate treatment. I met with both parents and asked them to allow Gabby to continue in treatment for a while longer in spite of the obvious progress she had made.

In the last 2 months of therapy, the child's tray was completely reversed (see Figure 2). Three-quarters of the tray was now occupied by Garfield, the giraffe, and the bear. The other quarter of the tray included four to six soldiers and tigers, separated from Garfield by a single fence, with no trees to facilitate climbing. "You know," I observed looking at the tray, "I think that Garfield is much safer now." "Yeah," Gabby replied, "the giraffe and the bear stay with her, and watch out for her." It was not necessary to say more. The healing had occurred in the sand work. There was no need for further interpretation.

I took three sessions to do termination work—two with Gabby alone and one that included her mother, father, and brother. During her last two sessions Gabby took out and "gave a bath" to all my miniatures and returned to her earlier play of filling up the cups with sand and pouring them out. When I told her that she would only be coming another two times, she didn't say much. I wondered what she would tell her mother about the termination, and when I inquired, Denise said that the night of the last meeting, right before going to sleep, Gabby had said, "I can go see Eliana when I want." Denise had told her she could, and Gabby had said, "Maybe some other time if my head aches."

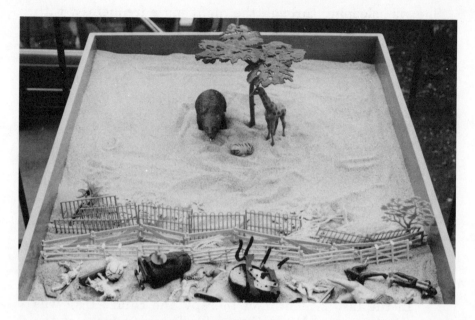

FIGURE 2

In the last session I talked to Gabby about when she had
first come to see me, reminding her that she had come in
slowly, with her mom, and hadn't played with too many
things in the playroom until later. I also reminded her that
at first she wanted her mom in the room, then mom was right
outside the door, and then mom waited with the other moms.
I also told Gabby that she had come to see me because I was
someone who talked to kids who had been hurt.

"I got hurt once," she said. "Those boys did bad things."

"Yes, they did, Gabby, and I'm sorry you got hurt."

"They got spanked, and their mommies were mad with
them and punished them."

"Yes Gabby, I bet that's so."

"But some boys are nice. Matt is nice."

"That's right, Gabby, lots of boys are nice."

Gabby played with the velcro darts and then remarked, "My mommy didn't know the bad kids came to my house."

"No Gabby. And your babysitter didn't know those boys would hurt you."

"They scared me," she said as her thumb found its way to her mouth.

"That was very scary, Gabby."

"They used to scare my nighttime."

"I remember, you used to have scary dreams." Gabby sat quietly and I asked her if she could draw a picture of the scary feeling. She grabbed the colors and made a picture full of black scribbles. Then I asked her to make a happy picture, and she drew a sun and a rainbow. I made a copy of each when she left. Gabby took her happy picture home but didn't want to take the scary one, telling me to keep it. Gabby ran back to the playroom to tell me, "My brother will kick their butts if they try to hurted me again." I assumed she had heard her brother say this, and then I summarized, "Your mom, dad, and brother—everyone who loves you—will take good care of you." "I know," she said. "My hurted is better now."

This was the most dialogue we had exchanged, and our last family meeting went very well. I said aloud, "When you brought Gabby to see me she had been hurt by those boys in the nighttime. She was very afraid, and all of you were worried for her, angry at the boys, and felt bad that you weren't there to take care of her." Denise and Gustavo instinctively added that they wished they had known what was going on; they would have come in and kept her safe. Matt added he'd kick anybody's butt who tried to hurt her again. Gabby giggled as Gustavo told Matthew to watch his language.

I noted that Gabby seemed to feel better now, safer, and that even though this was true, it was important that she knew that she could talk to her parents about the sexual abuse anytime she remembered it in the future. The parents again chimed in without prompting, reassuring her that she could always talk about how the boys had hurt her and ask any questions she had.

Finally, I asked Gabby if she and I could show everybody

her picture of the scary thing that happened. She grabbed it out of my hands, apparently pleased with the suggestion. She took it to her mother, father, and Matthew. I brought out some big easel paper and asked everyone to make a group picture of the bad thing that had happened to Gabby. They followed Gabby's lead and used colors rather than symbols. Then I asked them to draw a picture of a time when they all had a good time together, and they agreed on their vacation to Hawaii. (No one disillusioned Gabby by telling her that the vacation to Hawaii had not included her father, although the four of them had gone to Hawaii on a family vacation shortly after she was born.)

The family took approximately 5 minutes to draw the first picture and spent the remainder of the time working together on the family picture of Hawaii, drawing some tropical fish, which Gabby colored.

Before ending the session I asked the family to crumple up their drawing of the scary thing that had happened to Gabby and to throw it in a trash can I had brought to the center of the room. They passed the picture around, each one crumpling it more and more; then Matthew took the picture and jammed it into the trash can, imitating a Michael Jordan slam dunk. Gabby then asked where *her* scary picture was, crumpled it up herself, and mimicked her brother as she threw it into the can.

I told the family I was glad to have met them and been of assistance. I told Gabby she knew where I was if she ever wanted to come back and see me. She has never called, although she sent me a Valentine Day's card 2 years in a row.

DISCUSSION

The child's young age, specific symptomatology, and interest in sand tray therapy guided the therapy toward nondirective, nonintrusive play therapy.

Sand tray therapy is inherently self-healing and in this case was a miraculous process to watch. The child processed her trauma in her own way, at her own pace,

carefully symbolizing the overwhelming experience
through her play.

The sand tray illustrated her sense of entrapment and
feeling of defenselessness. She had felt isolated, without
internal or external resources to fight off her attackers. She
had been left afraid, hyperaroused, and avoidant of potentially threatening people and situations.

Certain issues that could be problematic were addressed
in the family session. Gabby heard and seemed to understand
that her parents did not know the boys were going to hurt
her and would have stopped them if they had known. A
termination ritual (with the drawings) symbolically empowered the family to place the past behind them and
negotiate for a safe future.

Gabby responded favorably to nondirective therapy, and
symbolically processed the trauma, while discharging her
feelings of fear and worry as she played in the sand. This
child also benefited greatly from having an appropriate family who followed therapeutic suggestions carefully.

Laurie: A Neglected Child Traumatized by a Hospitalization

REFERRAL INFORMATION

Laurie was a 7-year-old girl referred to me by her social worker for "reunification" treatment. Laurie, identified as a neglect victim, had been in foster care for the past year and a half while her parents completed a drug rehabilitation program in another county. Laurie had been returned to her biological parents 2 days before the social worker phoned me.

SOCIAL/FAMILY HISTORY

The social worker provided fragmentary information about the biological parents; the case had been transferred from another worker, and the records were in disarray. What was known is that prior to her placement in a foster home Laurie had been brought to an emergency room with appendicitis.

Her parents could not be found and were finally located after the child had been in the hospital for 4 days. The physician found Laurie to be a classic victim of neglect—undernourished, dirty, and suffering from minor infections, impetigo, and an untreated visual problem. Since the parents could not be located, the child was made a dependent of the court.

I met with both parents the day after the social worker's phone call and obtained a little more information. I found them to be guarded and slightly contentious. They immediately communicated their anger about being mandated into therapy. "We probably would have gone to counseling on our own," the father contended; he failed to understand the urgency of our appointment. The parents were also irate about having to pay for therapy and about the fact that Laurie was still a dependent of the court, overseen by a social worker for at least 6 months.

I reassured the parents that I understood all their complaints, and I quickly focused on how they felt about being reunited with Laurie after such a long separation. The parents slowly let down their guard and confided that they were afraid. They had been drug-free for a year and a half and had gone through daily counseling. They understood that they had been "less than perfect" parents and they seemed remorseful. When I inquired about their lives prior to the drug rehabilitation program, they described "hitting bottom," quickly adding, "The worse part of the whole thing is we dragged Laurie down with us." I remarked about the appropriateness of their concern for the child, and I told them that the more information I could get from them, the better I could help the child.

The parents described their history fleetingly and curtly. The father seemed to speak for the couple: "Both of us grew up with drunks as parents." He described how they had both been beaten and cast aside. The mother, Glenda, added that she had been useful to her family because she took care of her younger siblings. She said she had hated every minute of every day of her life and had quit school, running away with a drug-dealing boyfriend who used to sleep with her mother. Glenda commented, "I would say it was all downhill from there, but it was all downhill when I was brought home from the hospital." Glenda's drinking began at age 10, because sometimes there was little else to eat or drink around the house; she added, "when I drank was the only time I saw my mother laugh and look happy."

Laurie's father, Rob, likewise started drinking and smoking marijuana at a very early age. He said that he and his buddies would skip school, work on cars, and get stoned every day. His parents didn't care if he went to school or not. He was very proud of the fact that he could make good money working at a garage, and he now had a new job with an old employer who had taken a chance on him, as long as he stayed clean. Rob started living with his buddies in an abandoned shack when he was about 12 years old. "Remember the movie *Lost Boys*?" he asked. "That was what it was like."

I commented that both their lives seemed very unhappy and it was remarkable that they had taken such an important step in getting into a recovery program and committing themselves to staying sober. Mother said somberly, "Unfortunately, we had to hit bottom to get the message. I just hope Laurie isn't going to hate us for everything we did."

Both parents disavowed any contact with their biological parents. Glenda had a younger sister she kept in touch with but said she didn't care to see her mother or father ever again. Rob knew his father was alive, he would sometimes see him around, but, again, he seemed unmotivated to make contact. Both Glenda and Rob had truly rejected their own parents in an effort to escape their painful histories.

I asked the parents to describe the events that led to Laurie's being removed from them. They were visibly distressed as they spoke and had to take numerous cigarette breaks to endure the 2½-hour initial interview. They stated that they had been "heavily into the drug scene" since the time of Laurie's birth. Glenda said she made an effort to cut down on the drinking—but did drink throughout the pregnancy. Laurie was born underweight and fretful. She was kept in the hospital for weeks, and even then there were concerns about releasing her to her parents' care. A social worker and public health nurse visited for about 4 months;

the baby seemed to do pretty well except that she was difficult to feed and slept a lot.

Both parents stated that they had not planned to have a baby but liked the idea as soon as Laurie was born. Rob emphasized that he held a steady job and brought home enough money to feed the baby and buy diapers. He added that he and Glenda didn't eat too much in those days, so the money was just for Laurie.

The parents described Laurie as "quiet and really helpful" when she was older. Glenda said she was surprised that at the age of 5 the child could feed herself, go shopping at the store, and put herself to sleep watching TV. Rob said that Laurie liked to hang around the house: Even though she could come out with them when they went drinking, she preferred to stay at home. When I heard this, I spontaneously asked, "Did she stay home alone?" Noticing my concern, Glenda responded, "I know. Now when I think back on it, I can see how wrong that was. At the time, though, I thought I was being a good mom, letting her do what she wanted."

Glenda and Rob seemed earnestly concerned for the child and worried about the impact of their actions. They wanted to tell me the worst of what they had done. They described frequent drinking parties and said that drunks spent the night on Laurie's bed. Glenda became visibly distraught when she told me that some people had sex in their house; once she had walked into Laurie's room and found the child curled up in a corner crying while a couple was having sex on her bed.

Rob said that he had several drug-using friends and that Laurie had witnessed the use of needles and the snorting of cocaine. Sometimes people—including Glenda and Rob—passed out after taking drugs; the house was filthy because people used to vomit everywhere. Laurie was the one who tried to keep the place clean, her parents said, but it was really useless.

Glenda and Rob had been out drinking during Laurie's appendicitis. She had gone upstairs and had asked a neighbor for an aspirin. Neighbors noticed the child's fever and took her to the hospital (Laurie did not have a regular pediatrician, having had immunizations from the public health department and at school). When they talked about the appendicitis, both parents were in tears. Nevertheless, Rob added that it was the "best thing that ever happened to [them]."

I asked how much contact Rob and Glenda had had with Laurie during her placement. They said the contact was minimal; they had sent the social worker a few letters for Laurie, but they weren't sure she had received them.

When I asked them to describe Laurie during the last 2 days, they said she was really quiet and didn't smile much. "She was a little afraid of us at first," Rob said, "but she's beginning to warm up." The parents said that Laurie had been crying in her bed at night, so they had put her in their bed. When I commented that it was a good idea to let her get accustomed to her own room, Glenda agreed to do this on a temporary basis.

I reviewed with the parents what to tell Laurie about coming to see me. I told them this was a difficult time for all of them because they were, in fact, reconstructing a family, with few role models and few skills. They revealed that they were both attending AA meetings every day and had also joined a Parents Anonymous meeting to discuss parenting. Glenda asked if I knew where they could take classes, and I gave them a local resource, which they hesitated to contact. I also told them that I thought it would be beneficial for them to be in couples therapy to discuss the multitude of issues that would surface during these initial months. I referred them to a colleague for short-term therapy that would culminate in family therapy with the child.

Before the parents left, I asked them what they knew about Laurie's foster family and about how her separation from them had transpired. This was one area the parents had little insight into, and they seemed defensive. "I don't know, and I don't want to know," Rob said. "The social worker was trying to make some big deal about how Laurie would miss them, but I'm sure she's glad to be home." I stated that sometimes the children have two feelings at the same time when they go home: They're happy to see their parents and sad to leave the people who have been taking care of them. (I was careful not to use the term *foster parents* at this point, since this was obviously a sensitive topic.) Glenda seemed to understand this; Rob mumbled something under his breath.

CLINICAL IMPRESSIONS

Laurie was an extremely shy, slow moving, reticent, and compliant child. She was physically small, fragile-looking, very neat, and well groomed. There was a stark contrast between her pretty, bright, colorful dress, with bows along the edges of the skirt that matched the bows in her hair, and the somber, cautious look in her eyes and quiet mannerisms.

Laurie's hand was held by her mother. When Glenda removed her hand to do something, Laurie's arm dropped limply to her side. Mother held Laurie's hand again as they sat in the waiting room. I came out and introduced myself to the little girl, then took her on a tour of the playroom, indicating where we would be and where her mother would be. She offered no resistance as her mother prompted her to come with me.

Laurie looked around the playroom, thumb in mouth. I talked to her a little about the kinds of things she could play with. She wanted to color and sat at a little desk, coloring pages from a book. "Is it time to go yet?" became a standard question. At first I thought this indicated anxiety about being alone with me; I realized later that it was her desire to stay longer in this quiet, safe little place.

I decided to be very nondirective with this child. The parents had told me how they had tried to get her to tell them everything that had happened to her since they last had been together. I felt it was best to allow Laurie to come forward, rather than pressing in any way. I decided to sit next to her and do some coloring myself; as soon as I was engaged in my own activity, Laurie seemed to breathe easier.

The first four or five sessions followed suit. Laurie would enter the playroom quietly and engage in some coloring or reading activity. Because she had expressed a desire to read, I prominently displayed a book written for children in foster care called *Only One Oliver* (Rutter, 1978). This book talks about the loyalty issues felt by children who have warm feelings toward two sets of parents. Laurie read it quietly to herself a number of times. Then I asked, "You were in foster care, weren't you, Laurie?"

"Uh, huh," she said.

"Who did you live with?"

"Jack and Leona and Steffi and Harry."

"Who are they?"

"My mom...foster mom and dad and my...the other kids who lived there."

"Do you think about them sometimes?"

"Uh, Hum."

"How does that make you feel, to miss them?"

"I don't know," she said as she turned away. We had made a beginning.

THE BEGINNING PHASE OF TREATMENT

Once she was familiar with the environment and the structure and could tolerate talking with me, Laurie seemed to relax. In addition, she was obviously more comfortable with her mother than she had been when I first met her, as reflected by her posture and flexibility in the waiting room.

Laurie slowly made her way over to the dollhouse and began some play involving a mother, father, and three children. My hypothesis was that she was recreating the foster home, not her current home. She had the mother cook breakfast and make sure the children had clean clothes; the father watched TV when he came home from work. The family laughed when the father told jokes; they would frequently prepare a picnic basket and go outside to play ball. Laurie said that she was a good "catcher," and when I told her I had a ball in the playroom, she asked me to throw to her and she would catch. She greatly enjoyed this activity, apparently reminiscent of happier times. "Jack is the bestest catcher; he taught me how to catch," she said loudly.

The parents' therapist and I had been in touch: She was

disheartened by their continued failure to understand the child's feelings toward her foster parents. Glenda and Rob had forbidden Laurie to mention the foster parents' names and had become very distressed when Laurie inadvertently referred to the foster mother as "Mom." The parents' therapist felt that they held the foster parents in some way responsible for their not seeing their child for almost 2 years and that this illogical view did not allow for other perceptions. After the first month of therapy I made an appointment with the foster parents and I asked the parents to attend. Rob and Glenda were furious that I felt it necessary to talk to "those people" but felt they had to attend the meeting.

The meeting was tense and awkward for the first half hour. Glenda and Rob had been 15 minutes late, and I was afraid to start without them. When they arrived I expressed my delight at seeing them and made an opening statement regarding the purpose of the meeting: "As I've told Laurie's parents, I wanted to meet with you, Leona and Jack, so you could tell us how Laurie was during the time she was in your home." Leona and Jack, obviously real professionals, immediately reassured Laurie's parents. "We are so glad to meet you. We found Laurie a real delight. She was so well behaved and so sweet. When a child is like that, you know they've had some good parents." Glenda and Rob looked shocked and couldn't find a response; they looked at each other and held hands. Rob talked first, as usual: "Did she have any problems at your house?" Leona and Jack described a passive, compliant, helpful child. They portrayed these as positive behaviors, yet I knew they were communicating the child's weaknesses as well. "Sometimes you hardly knew she was there—she would melt into the woodwork." I had often heard this phrase used to describe abused or neglected children who learn to stay safe by staying out of the way.

Jack and Leona said they were an active family; they took frequent trips to parks, lakes, and camping sites. They said Laurie loved the outdoors and was good at hiking, running, swimming, and playing ball. Glenda said quietly, "I didn't know she could swim." Laurie's foster parents said they had taught her to swim because the doctors had suggested she resume normal activity after her surgery. Since they didn't know what she liked, they thought they would try swimming.

Rob wanted to know if she ever asked about him or Glenda. The foster parents quickly exchanged glances, and Jack answered, "She would talk about both of you often, saying how you used to have big parties and had lots of friends." Jack added, "We also talked to her about her mommy and daddy too, letting her know what a good thing you were doing getting some help with your problem." Jack, himself a recovering alcoholic, made an astonishing divulgence: "Rob, I know firsthand what it's like. I have 15 years recovery, and every day I remind myself how far down I got before I could pull myself up."

Whatever antagonism, jealousy, or displaced anger existed before was dissipated during this meeting. Both sets of parents went out for coffee and, miraculously, Rob and Glenda invited Jack and Leona to come over for dinner. Laurie came in excitedly the following week and told me Jack and Leona were coming over to see her. She was plainly thrilled and, fortunately, she no longer felt she had to keep her excitement under tap.

Treatment Plan

After the first month I made a treatment plan consisting of individual treatment and conjoint family sessions:

1. Individual treatment
   a. Use nondirective play therapy sessions to establish a strong therapeutic alliance.
   b. Document play themes (e.g., foster care separation).
   c. Become directive by talking about her life with her biological parents, now and then.
   d. Discuss her surgery.
2. Conjoint family sessions
   a. Discuss structural issues such as boundaries, privacy, limits.

    b. Discuss parenting issues such as discipline, guidance, and fun activities.

    c. Discuss how family members feel about being reunited and what problems they have encountered.

    d. Make sure child has regular medical care, updated immunization plans, and that family has nutritional counseling.

3. Coordination

    a. Discuss a plan for contact with foster parents.

    b. Talk to school personnel about Laurie's school performance and behavior.

    c. Contact social worker about dependency issue.

THE MIDDLE PHASE OF TREATMENT

I asked Laurie to draw me a picture of herself, and she made a very small, very faint picture of a little girl with no hands and feet and a hole in the middle (Figure 1). When I asked her to draw a picture of her family, she made several attempts, erased them, and seemed very frustrated. Sensing her dilemma, I asked, "Which family do you want to draw first?" "I don't know," she responded, "I'm not a good drawer." "I think you're a fine drawer," I stated and took the initiative. "I know what—since Glenda and Rob were your first family,

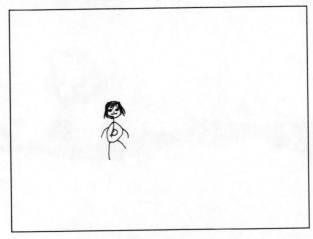

FIGURE 1

draw them first." As can be seen in Figure 2, Laurie drew her mother lying down and her father watching TV. There is no structure or foundation in the drawing, and it seems as though the figures are floating. The disparity between this drawing and Figure 3, a drawing of Jack and Leona, is striking. Not only is the latter picture more detailed but it has emotional content and contact between family members. The foster home had clearly been an emotionally rewarding and nurturing environment for the child.

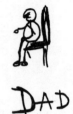

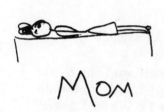

FIGURE 2

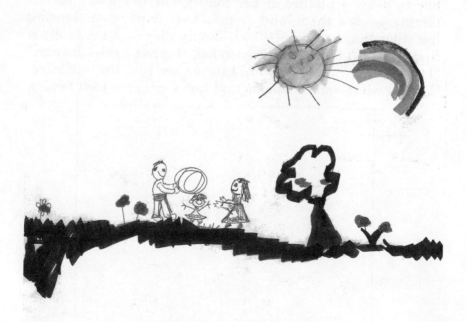

FIGURE 3

Laurie had relaxed in the therapy hour (and, from the parents' reports, had become more relaxed in the home setting as well). She was more talkative and directed her play well. She would choose the dollhouse frequently—to show her "ideal" family. She would ask me to throw the ball; she felt competent and proud as her catching skills improved. When she began throwing the ball into the hoop, she couldn't wait to show her foster father what she had learned. Although she talked about her parents in a guarded fashion, it appeared that all Laurie's associations with fun or recreation had to do with the foster parents. (I talked to her parents' therapist about helping them plan a weekend picnic or trip, and they had been responsive.)

Soon Laurie's own self-portrait began to change (Figure 4), gaining in size and accuracy. Her schoolwork was going well, and she always made a point of telling me how her mother helped her with her homework. (I verified that this was the case and not just the child's unfulfilled wish.)

The therapy shifted one day when Laurie made her self-portrait and I noticed that the middle part of her picture

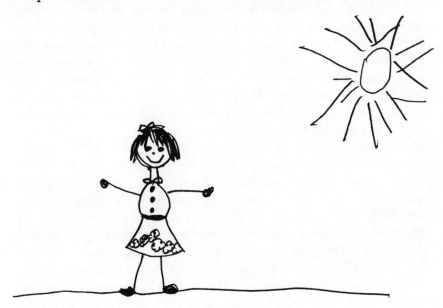

FIGURE 4

looked different. "It's getting better," she said, adding quickly, "I can hardly feel it anymore." She was referring to her
surgery, and I seized the opportunity. I brought down some
toys of hospital equipment from the shelf and showed them
to her; they became her primary source of play for the next
eight sessions. Each week Laurie would scurry in, ask for the
boxes with the hospital equipment, and enact an elaborate
scenario, including a ride in an ambulance, a hospital operating room, and a recovery room. She would bring a girl doll to
the hospital, get her into surgery, and give her jello and soup
in the recovery room. Immediately after surgery she would
wrap the girl doll in tissue and with a red felt-tip pen she
would put some red dots on the tissue. "It's bleeding...she's
not well yet," she explained.

Affectively, Laurie was constricted and robot-like during
this play. During the surgery itself she was perfectly still and
appeared worried and afraid. In the recovery room she looked
sad and lonely, and, finally, when the play was over, she
would play catch with me, apparently in an effort to make
herself feel better.

Glenda and Rob called because Laurie had been having
some nightmares and was sucking her thumb again. I reassured them that she was doing fine and that we were working
on some painful memories. "About us?" the parents asked,
with their characteristic defensiveness. "No," I responded,
"it's about her surgery." When I asked if they had noticed any
other unusual behavior, they said she had lost her appetite
and was complaining of a stomachache.

Laurie's posttraumatic play was triggering off a number
of regressed behaviors. The play was repetitive, and Laurie's
anxiety remained constant. At the ninth session I decided to
intervene, since the anxiety generated in the play was apparently having some negative repercussions on the child.
My first intervention was to provide a commentary on events
throughout the play. Laurie seemed almost shocked at first
but gradually seemed to pace her play so that I had a chance
to describe each sequence. "The little girl is put in an ambulance. I bet the ambulance goes fast, and I bet there's a
siren." "No," she said, "their siren was broken that day." "Oh,"
I continued, "the ambulance with the broken siren is going

very fast. The little girl has a stomachache...." "And a headache," Laurie editorialized. I would incorporate Laurie's own comments and continue narrating the events. I finished with "The little girl is in her own room now, eating soup and jello and getting stronger every day." "Yeah," Laurie added. When I said, "I wonder how this little girl feels eating her jello and soup," Laurie did not respond.

She repeated this play the following week. A noticeable addition occurred: Laurie responded to the last question about the little girl's feelings by saying, "I think she's scared and lonely." "Oh," I said, "the little girl is feeling afraid and lonely as her body gets stronger and heals." When Laurie nodded, I continued: "I wonder why she might feel afraid." Laurie softly added, "She doesn't know where her mommy and daddy are." "Oh," I agreed, "not knowing where your mommy and daddy are would be a really scary thing."

In the following weeks, using this basic approach, Laurie was able to talk about the feelings she had while she was recuperating in the hospital: worrying about her parents; not knowing who was feeding a stray cat she looked after; being scared about the shots, the tube in her arm, the stitches that had to come out; and not knowing where she would go when she left the hospital. "Ooooh," I said, "that's a lot to worry about. Was there anybody who you could talk with?" "No...wait, yeah. A nice lady came to see me." I checked the hospital records and found that a hospital counselor had been to see Laurie every other day. Once she had come with the social worker to tell Laurie that they had found a new home for her where she would stay until they knew where her parents were. Laurie seemed to suddenly remember: "The lady came to tell me when they found Mom and Dad, and she told me they were going to go to the hospital to get better from their drinking problem."

The second level of intervention was to review the sequence of events in Laurie's play scenario and interject some mechanism for releasing affect as we went along. For example, when the girl doll was in the ambulance, I asked Laurie to "put the little girl's feelings into words." I prompted, "What is she feeling right now?" "She's really scared," Laurie answered, "Not just a little, either." This method revealed that Laurie thought she had done something wrong and was being taken away to be punished.

The third stage came when I began to call the girl doll "Laurie" instead of saying "the little girl." Laurie didn't flinch or question this change.

And then, as a final elaboration of her play, I had Laurie speak to the ambulance people, the doctors, the "nice lady" counselor, the social worker, and her parents. When I first directed her to speak to her parents, she froze. "I can't," she said.

"What would happen if you did?"

"Maybe they would get mad."

"And what do they say or do when they're mad?"

"I don't know."

"Have you ever seen them mad?"

"No," she answered, and this was likely true, based on the parents' description of themselves as "mellow, sleepy drunks." I told her that she could speak for Laurie, and I would answer for her parents. She seemed to like that, unaware that when I came to my part of the roleplay, I would take a helpless position and ask her for direction. At times she was unable to speak; I would instruct her to take deep breaths, move her arms, jump up and down, and then I would inquire again.

When she spoke as Laurie for the first time, she cried and sucked her thumb. "Why did you go away?" she sobbed. "I did something bad, didn't I?" And finally, "Did you want me to die?" I let her cry for a long time and sat next to her quietly. Laurie held her big bunny tightly and rocked a little in place. Her questions were so heartfelt and basic. When I asked how I, playing the part of her parents, should respond, she didn't know. Feeling I should refrain from "fixing things" immediately, I said, "You know, Laurie, I bet your mom and dad would like to answer these questions. How would it be if we had them come in with you one day, and we could give them a chance to explain." Laurie seemed hesitant and yet willing. "I can't cry if they come," she said. "How come?" I asked. "What will happen if you do?" "They'll feel bad," she stated, reflecting her characteristic caretaker role. "Sometimes, Laurie," I explained, "it's OK to feel bad for mistakes we've made. Everyone makes mistakes and feels bad later."

We played catch for a little while, and when we went to the waiting room at the end of the therapy session, I told Laurie's mother that Laurie and I would like to invite her and Rob to meet with us. Glenda, knowing this would eventually happen, seemed resigned and nervous. We set a tentative time for the following week.

The parents' therapist prepared them for the meeting. Glenda and Rob seemed eager to clarify any concerns Laurie may have felt about being unloved. During the meeting they were exceptional in their ability to be open, reassure the child, and allow themselves to cry in front of Laurie and yet relieve her of the need to offer any caretaking responses. Their years of counseling had paid off: They were appropriate and very nurturing. The parents had complained about their child's lack of physical response to their hugs and kisses; this was the first time Laurie clung to them both as they engulfed her with a caring hug.

And as comforting and as necessary as this work was, I brought up yet another difficult emotion: anger. "Laurie," I said, "I'm really glad that your mom and dad have answered your questions." I had given her many opportunities to ask additional questions and make other statements she wanted. "One more thing I just want you all to think about is that when things like this happen, even when there are good explanations, the person who has felt scared or lonely can also feel angry at the people who went away." Laurie buried her head in her father's shoulder. Rob picked up on what I was saying immediately and said, "That's right, honey. You have every right to feel mad at us, not only because we left you at home alone and you got sick but also because we had to be separated when we went to the hospital and you went to Leona and Jack's house. It's OK for you to feel mad about that. I would if I were you." Laurie smiled as her dad tickled her a little, but I knew that the last stage of therapy would concentrate on this more difficult emotion.

Indeed, the work that remained was difficult and painful. Not only was I working with Laurie on her anger but the parents' therapist reported that Glenda was working on her immense guilt over drinking while pregnant. Father was processing the guilt he had at putting his child at such risk from drug dealers and "sex perverts."

Meanwhile, the family developed a good relationship with the foster parents. At first, because of too flexible boundaries, Rob and Glenda had spent too much time with the foster family. At their therapist's suggestion, they made a commitment to get together no more than once a month. That way, Laurie could make her transition more easily.

Laurie's status as a dependent of the court was terminated at the 6-month review of her case, with recommendations for this action from both the parents' and child's therapists.

When therapy was terminated, after a total of 9 months, I made an exception to my rule about toys not leaving the playroom and gave the little girl doll to Laurie. I told her that the little doll would be a reminder of all the work we had done on her thoughts and feelings during a very difficult time. The parents later told me that the little girl doll had been prominently displayed in Laurie's room and that they had frequently spotted Laurie discussing her feelings with the doll. Immediately following termination of the therapy, I had told Laurie she could call me if she wanted to say hello or talk. She had called a couple of times just to say hello, and I had received Christmas and Thanksgiving cards from her.

The parents called me 2 years after termination asking for some help for a sexual problem in their relationship. I referred them to a sex therapist and inquired about Laurie. She had become a member of a swim team, was doing very well in school, and had responded with ambivalence to the news of a new brother or sister.

DISCUSSION

Laurie was a 7-year-old child recently reunited with severely neglecting parents. She had lived in a foster home for the past year and a half, while her parents successfully participated in a drug rehabilitation program. Laurie had survived in her neglectful home by becoming pseudomature and caretaking her parents. She had initially been extremely worried for them when they could not be found and had suffered severe loneliness when she underwent surgery without them.

Laurie was regressed, had difficulty making attachments, appeared lethargic, and was seemingly depressed and unresponsive. During treatment her strong bond to the foster family became clear, and an intervention was made to advance a proper separation from the foster parents. Laurie had apparently made a positive attachment to the foster parents, enjoying family outings and partaking in physical activity previously unknown to her. She felt acute loyalty conflicts between her foster parents and biological parents, having concrete positive memories of the foster home and abstract negative memories of her own family.

In therapy Laurie engaged in posttraumatic play once she was exposed to some hospital toys in my office. She ritualistically acted out her fear, worry, and loneliness. She had interpreted her parents' absence during her hospitalization as a complete rejection and punishment for imagined wrongs she had committed. After being reunited with her parents Laurie was reserved about physical contact with them until she heard directly from their mouths the answers to all her questions about their abandonment of her.

Laurie's posttraumatic play produced great anxiety, manifested by her labored movement, constricted breathing, and facial rigidity. There were occasions during the play when she shook and appeared to perspire. I intervened in the posttraumatic play by verbally depicting each sequence, allowing Laurie to correct my commentary. It seems that these interventions had the effect of enabling her to observe, while experiencing and processing difficult and frightening negative feelings associated with the traumatic event. At the same time, because she was having the troubling feelings while she was in a safe setting, it was easier for her to separate the past from the present. As Laurie observed and helped me verbalize what had happened to "the little girl" in the ambulance, I shifted to asking about *her* feelings and thoughts, not the little girl's. She responded immediately, sharing some of what she remembered about her hospitalization. The props, detailed as they are, allowed her to remember many things she might otherwise have forgotten (like how bright the lights were in the operating room and how white the hospital gowns were).

In her play Laurie was able to cry, seemingly recreating her sense of loneliness. This affect led to verbalizations that clearly reflected the worries she had had in the hospital about being bad, unworthy, and rejected. The family sessions were momentous for this child. Rather than giving in to the temptation to answer her questions during the play, I told Laurie that I would help her to share her feelings with her parents directly.

This child suffered considerable damage from extremely neglectful parents who had placed her at great risk of abuse from others. She had been exposed to explicit sexual behavior of adults and had frequently been left to fend for herself. The parents continued marital and family therapy; the year and a half in a drug treatment program had been invaluable. They faced many painful feelings of guilt and shame and were very committed to helping repair the damage done to their child.

Sharlene: A Child Traumatized by Severe Sexual Abuse

REFERRAL INFORMATION

Sharlene, an 8-year-old girl, was referred to treatment upon the advice of a social worker. Sharlene had been placed in a foster home when she was removed from her natural father at age 5. The foster parents had noticed some "bizarre" behaviors and wanted the child seen by a professional. Sharlene had previously been in counseling for a year and a half; her counselor had since died.

SOCIAL/FAMILY HISTORY

The police reports and court documents painted a bleak picture of Sharlene's life. Her mother died from a drug overdose when the child was 2 years old. Nothing is known about Sharlene's mother or her level of care for the child. The natural father, Walter, was a convicted felon who had been incarcerated for numerous drug possession charges. He had also been charged with aggravated assault at a younger age.

The child was discovered at the age of 5 years through pornographic pictures that were developed at a local camera shop. Required to report suspected child abuse, the camera shop owner gave police the photographs of Sharlene in numerous sexual positions with a variety of men.

Apparently, Walt was not a child molester himself but served as a kind of pimp for his 4-year-old daughter. He had made a large sum of money selling the pictures of his child having sex with adults. Aside from keeping her well fed and photogenic, her father had no apparent regard for Sharlene's well-being. In addition to the photographs, the police uncovered videotapes in which the child, appearing drugged, was penetrated by adolescent boys. Several videotapes showed her performing fellatio on adolescent boys, riding them cowboy-style in the nude, and having cherries and candies sucked out of her vagina.

Needless to say, this child had been severely sexually abused; her initial treatment focused on the symptomatic sexualized behavior she had developed, which included excessive masturbation. In addition, upon placement, Sharlene had suffered from nightmares, somnambulism, and unprovoked outbursts of anger and emotionality. She was virtually nonverbal and developmentally delayed; she had very few social skills, frequently stripping her clothes off, even in public places.

The foster parents, Ann and Phillip, had expressed an interest in and a willingness to adopt the child. They had no children of their own and wanted to eventually adopt two more children.

When I met with Ann and Phillip, I affirmed the appropriateness of the referral. Sharlene was doing well in many ways, yet they had observed bizarre behaviors, best summarized as follows:

1. Trance-like behaviors
2. Forgetfulness and denial of observed behavior
3. Sporadic amnesia for the abuse

4. Fluctuations in ability
5. Self-mutilation
6. Hurting animals
7. Using another name
8. Fluctuations and polarizations in behavior

THE BEGINNING PHASE OF TREATMENT

Sharlene was an overweight, appealing child who appeared older than her 8 years of age. She dressed in a provocative manner, resembling a teenager more than a latency-age child.

Sharlene entered treatment easily, almost eagerly. She asked where my playroom was and seemed indifferent to her foster mother and where she would remain. She inspected the playroom aggressively, opening things, taking things out of containers, and throwing things aside to get to something she wanted. Uncharacteristically, I laid out all the rules of the playroom right away. "That's cool," she said as she continued her exploration of the room. She had a tremendous amount of energy and spoke almost nonstop.

"Do you know why your mom has brought you to counseling?" I asked.

"She's not my mom. She's my adoptive mom," she asserted. This was interesting since I had asked her foster mother what labels were used at home and she told me that Sharlene had called them "Mommy" and "Daddy" almost immediately.

"What do you usually call her?" I asked.

"Annie," she responded. "That's what Phil calls her."

"Oh," I persevered, "and what did Phil and Annie tell you about coming to counseling?"

She took a big breath, "They said I have to come here because they're worried 'cause I forget things a lot."

"What do you think?" I inquired.

"I think that's for me to know and you to find out."

I smiled and said, "OK...you've just met me; I guess you'll feel like talking more as you know me better." I realized quickly that whatever I said, Sharlene disagreed with it.

"Nah, no problem. I don't need more time. I forget lots of things. Like sometimes they say I said something I didn't."

"Give me an example," I directed.

"Well, like yesterday. Annie got bent out of shape because she said that I had told her I wasn't getting any new books in school. Well, I know I didn't say that because I got to get some new books, it's the beginning of the year."

"Do you usually forget things that you say?"

"I don't know...I forgot," she said and laughed heartily in my face.

"You've got a sense of humor," I noted.

Then she responded, "Phil said I took my bike out for a ride and got a flat tire...it wasn't me; I don't like to ride my stupid old bike."

Sharlene found a game of Chinese checkers and, setting it down on the floor, said, "I used to beat my old doctor all the time. You want to bet money?" I replied, "Nope. No money for me. But let's set them up; I'll take blue." As I said that she took the blue for herself and gave me the reds; "Too late, too late, I already picked the blue," she said. Every time Sharlene advanced she teased me about being behind. Every time she got a new marble into the triangle, she danced around the room, saying, "I'm going to skunk you, I'm going to skunk you."

My exhaustion was only matched by her apparent surge in enthusiasm as she left my office, announcing loudly that she had beaten the pants off of me—an interesting choice of words. As they left the first session Ann remarked that Sharlene wasn't always so loud.

The following session I observed a markedly changed child. Sharlene's clothing was subdued, and her manner was constrained and gentle. She didn't seem to remember much about the playroom, asking if certain things had been there the week before. When I asked her what she remembered about the previous session, she said she remembered that I was a little fat and that we had played a game on the floor. She couldn't remember the name of the game, and when I reminded her, she said she didn't know how to play Chinese checkers but liked to color. She made some attempts at a tree and flowers, chastising herself for being unartistic. While she was coloring, I asked her what she thought about my being a little fat.

"Oh, I didn't mean to hurt your feelings."

"You didn't," I said. "I was just wondering what you thought about it."

"Some kids at school would laugh at you."

"How come?" I asked.

"Because you're a little fat."

"Oh," I remarked, "does that happen to kids that are a little fat at school?"

"Yeah," she said quietly, "it hurts my feelings when they laugh at me."

"I can understand your feelings being hurt." I paused, then asked, "How do you feel when your feelings are hurt?"

"I feel like crying a lot, but I won't," she said in a declarative voice.

"What would happen if you cried?" I asked.

Sharlene looked up at me and said, "If I start crying, I'm scared I may never stop."

"Oh," I said, "That's an interesting thought."

"I know. I have lots of funny ideas."

I realized that using the word *interesting* might have sounded strange to Sharlene. I tried to expand on the meaning by saying, "I've heard other kids say that sometimes, that they get worried they may cry forever."

She looked up in shock. "Somebody else said that?" she asked with intense interest.

"Yeah."

"What happened to her?"

"Well," I replied, taking my time, "she had lots of things to cry about, and found she could cry a little at a time."

Sharlene began to draw a picture of a little girl, her tears being caught in little cups. "See," she said, "she cried little bits at a time." "Yeah," I said, "you got a picture of that in your mind, and now you drew it out. You're pretty smart." "That's what my mom says," she reported, as she stood up and began to look around. She found the baby dolls and changed their clothes, bathed them, and combed their hair. "I like it here," she commented and seemed disappointed that the timer's bell marked the end of the session. I sat bewildered for a few minutes, understanding the parents' concerns.

In the third and fourth sessions, Sharlene played with the dolls exclusively, repeatedly dressing and undressing them, diapering them, bathing them, feeding them, and combing their hair. My treatment plan revealed the exploratory nature of the treatment to date:

1. Individual play therapy
    a. Observe fluctuations in behavior.
    b. Have weekly contact with parents re. child's behavior at home.
    c. Be nondirective.
    d. Provide art materials; she uses them well.
2. Coordination
    a. Talk to teachers about her behavior at school.
    b. Obtain copies of the police report.
    c. Ascertain legal status of Walter.
3. Working hypothesis
    a. Assess for dissociative disorders.
    b. Assess for multiple personality disorder (MPD).

The fifth and sixth sessions changed drastically. Sharlene behaved in a manner identical to that displayed in her first visit, playing in a chaotic way, choosing many games she would start and not finish, and being loud and disruptive. These sessions reflected her internal disorganization. I asked Sharlene's foster parents how the week had been and learned that her difficult behavior at home was consistent with the chaotic therapy sessions. (I also learned that the 3 sessions in which she had been calm and soft-spoken had coincided with good weeks at home.)

My plan was to have the quieter Sharlene draw me a self-portrait the next time she was available. In the following session I seized the opportunity, and Sharlene drew a faint little person on a bed in the middle of the page. She folded it up and said that was all the drawing she wanted to do for today. When she came back for her sessions over the following three weeks, she unfolded her piece of paper and added another drawing to it (see Figure 1). As she made her draw-

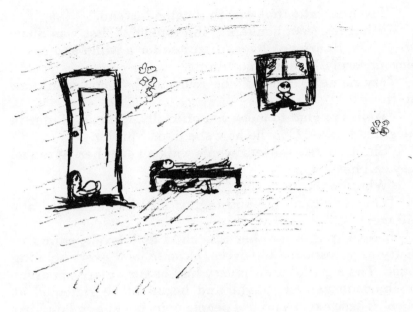

FIGURE 1

ings I would ask, "Who's that?" and "What's she or he doing?"
The first figure drawn (the child in the bed in the center) she
would not speak about. The second figure (a child in a window
with big eyes) she said was "Chuck, a boy who is watching to
make sure no bad people come." The third figure (a little
person in a closet) was Marsha ("she's little and she's
pretending to be dead"). The fourth figure (a person under a
bed) was "Linda," who was really mad and was going to kill
Daddy." Since no other figures were added to the drawings,
I asked again about the first one, and this time Sharlene said,
"That's Josie and she likes what the bad men do to her."
Sharlene always folded up this drawing carefully and stored
it in a box that we set high up on a shelf in the corner of the
playroom so no one could see it. This reflected the child's
ambivalence about visibility.

The next time the loud Sharlene came, I welcomed her
and brought out the Chinese checkers. We sat and played,
and I commented, "Did you come to therapy last week?"

"Nope...I had things to do."

"I wonder who that was that came instead."

"What are you, bonkers?" she replied, "That was Sharlene." "Oh, Sharlene...I see." I waited for a while and asked very sincerely, "What's *your* name?"

"My name's Charlie," she responded. "Don't you know anything?"

"Well, I'm glad to meet you officially, Charlie." Later in the game I asked Charlie how she liked Sharlene.

"She's a bore...she lets people walk all over her. At school they call her a wimp."

"What do they call you?" I asked.

"They don't call me nothing, or I'll kick their ass," she told me.

It appeared to me that this child had developed multiplicity as a response to severe, chronic, and overwhelming abuse. The signs of multiplicity had become more apparent as Sharlene gained weight and began to be ridiculed at school. These experiences of people pointing at her, laughing at her, and hurting her feelings had caused enough stress to create or stimulate fragmented parts of her personality or "alters," probably created to defend against the sexual abuse. Sharlene's self-portrait had been telling in that she had portrayed herself as all the different characters of her personality. Since it appeared that the divergent parts were little, I suspected that they had originated during the years of abuse, when Sharlene was small.

The key seemed to lie in the self-portrait. Sharlene's next session gave us a chance to talk more about it. Sharlene went to the box on the shelf to pull out her drawing; unfolding it, she seemed eager to review it with me, as had become her habit. In previous sessions I would ask her questions about the drawing, but this time, when she told me about the different parts of herself ("alters"), I inquired about their ages and if they had other names they used. When we got to Chuck, Sharlene said in a matter-of-fact way that Chuck sometimes called himself Charlie. When I asked what she knew about Charlie, Sharlene said that he was "tough and strong" and liked to take care of people. During this session, I took a chance and made the following statement to Sharlene: "Sharlene, is this a picture of you?" She calmly folded up the picture, stored it away, and waited for the session to end. Charlie appeared at the next two sessions. When Sharlene returned, she once again took out the picture. I asked again, "Sharlene, is this a picture of you?"

"I think so," she said.

"Some children who have been hurt very badly, have lots of different parts that make up who they are."

"Do you know the bad things that happened to me?" she asked bewildered.

"Yes, Sharlene, your foster mom told me."

"OOOh," she said, "I don't like people to know that."

"What will they think?"

"They'll think I'm bad."

I controlled my instinct to reassure her and responded, "It's really hard to think people think you're bad. You have to remember that when you got hurt, you were a little kid, and it was the grown-ups who did something wrong, not you."

A little tear appeared. "I sort of liked some of it," she said.

"That's OK too." I needed to give her some information: "Sometimes kids who get hurt sexually talk about how their bodies felt good or some of the games were fun."

"Marty told me I did it the best of anybody."

"Did what?"

"You know."

"I'm not sure what you mean."

Sharlene, in her sweet little voice, said, "sucked him off." She looked away, but I couldn't tell if she was embarrassed or scared or pleased she had spoken.

"Sharlene, everybody likes to be told they do something better than anybody else. You're not bad because you like to do something well." She had said and heard enough, and she looked at the timer. "What was it like to talk about what happened to you?"

"Well, I guess it was OK."

I told Sharlene that my job was to talk to kids about their thoughts and feelings and that there wasn't anything she could say that would scare me or make me think she was bad. I think that was the wrong thing to say because Charlie came in with a chip on his/her shoulder the next session, calling me a slew of bad names and testing all my limits. At one point during the session he/she reached between my legs and grabbed my genitals firmly. I removed his/her hand and said, "Charlie, it's not OK for you to touch private parts of my body, and I won't touch private parts of your body. I'm sure you're trying to find out if this is OK, because other grown-ups you've known have asked to be touched or have touched you. For me, this is not OK to do. Any questions?" Charlie mumbled, "Yeah, yeah, you prude," but I knew I had made my point. I had responded swiftly and nonpunitively and had set a clear limit. Sharlene was showing me the "bad" part of herself, and I did not reject her or punish her.

Sharlene came to therapy for the next 3 months. She was much more comfortable talking about the abuse and, in fact, began some posttraumatic play that lasted for over 3 months.

I was now in a much more directive phase of treatment, and it appeared that Sharlene needed acceptance and active engagement, information, and assistance in acknowledging and expressing her feelings. She found an unused silk pillow with a shiny surface and placed a Barbie doll in the center of the pillow, posing her in a variety of suggestive positions, including explicit sexual play with the Ken doll and with other male dolls. She used a toy camera to take pictures and play the part of the director. Thus, Sharlene was acting out the role of her father, Walt, and had chosen the Barbie doll to represent herself.

During this play Sharlene would always have a bowl and spoon handy and she would do something that resembled dissolving a pill and force-feeding it to the Barbie doll. Sometimes Barbie resisted swallowing the medicine, but most of the time she complied. Walt was alternately menacing and kind: He would offer Barbie milk-shakes and candy if she did what she was told; other times he threatened to whip her "shapely little butt" if she didn't cooperate.

The Barbie doll made grunting sounds resembling an adult woman enjoying sex; Sharlene also forced the doll's pelvis up and down, making suggestive adult comments. When I asked how she knew to do that, she said Walt had shown her lots of movies of women having sex. Her knowledge of sexual toys and positions seemed endless, and she had learned the most crude descriptive terms. During these sessions Sharlene was obviously aroused, and I was concerned about the reinforcement of arousal to these negative sexual experiences. I was also concerned about my own observer role, since many individuals had apparently witnessed her sexual exploitation.

I decided, therefore, to intervene in the ritualized play. "Where are the different parts of you, Sharlene?" She replied, "That's a good idea; I'll put them out." She selected dolls to represent the different parts of herself, and situated them near the central scene of the play. "Let's have Chuckie talk to the cameraman," I said. Sharlene seemed irritated by my interrupting her play, yet she agreed and placed the Chuck doll in her hand. "Hey, Walt. Hey butthead," she screamed out. "If you have to be so secretive about this, it must be really wrong. I'm tired of you making me stand guard. I'm tired of being your guard." She intuitively and immediately assumed the personality of Marsha, whom she had earlier drawn as the little girl in the closet, and said in a weak and miserable little voice, "Walt, can't you hear me...I'm dying here. I'm not going to be around to make your movies anymore. I'm dying here, can you hear me?" Sharlene threw down the doll and went out of the office. I caught up with her, but she wanted to leave. She had done more than she could. I sat with her outside for a while, looking at the flowers and a spider's nest and letting her show me how she could jump rope.

I reminded myself about pacing. This child was now entering the trauma, and the associated feelings of despair, fear, and helplessness were entering the treatment hour. She had apparently resisted coming to therapy the following week, and her foster mother called to report that she was sick. I talked to her briefly on the phone, telling her that we were talking about some really hard memories right now and it was OK for her to take a little break. When she came back, I assured her, we would take it a little at a time.

The play ceased spontaneously at this point, but Sharlene wanted to use her drawings to act out the various parts.

Eventually, I asked her to have Charlie talk to some of the other alters and encouraged the alters to interact with each other. I also talked to the alters about the feelings *they* held and asked for them by name when I did. Only the catatonic alter (the child pretending to be dead in the drawing) refused to come out and talk to me directly; I realized later that even though Sharlene had tried to role-play this part of her personality, this alter was nonverbal.

I had begun to see Charlie less in therapy; I asked Sharlene if I could show the self-portrait to Charlie, and she agreed. "He won't like it," she said. "He doesn't like anything that I do."

"Why do you think that is?" I inquired.

"Because...he thinks I'm wimpy."

"I think he worries about you and wants you to take care of yourself better. He wants to make sure no one hurts you. He's there just to help you."

Sharlene seemed to like this idea and said, "Yeah, like my bodyguard."

"Yeah," I repeated, "just like a bodyguard, but he wishes you didn't need one."

"I get it," she announced.

I showed Charlie the self-portrait and she/he was unimpressed. "She doesn't draw very well."

"I think she draws fine. Do you know who these people are?"

"Yep, the slut, the goonie, and the dyke." Charlie was so cryptic. I asked further and learned that he called the little girl who wanted to die a "goonie" because he thought that was less than a wimp. He called the sexualized girl "the slut" but said "she didn't know any better...women are stupid." He called the aggressive one "the dyke," his way of referring to strong women. I assumed he had learned these judgmental concepts from Walt. "What do you call yourself?" I asked. "They call me Chuck," he replied. "Yeah," I persisted, "but what do you call yourself?" I had never seen him drop the facade as he did this one time, stating concisely, "Rambo." That pretty much summed it up. This alter had been created to try to fight unbeatable odds on his own, just as Rambo had done with armies. "You and I are going to need to teach Sharlene how to be more assertive and not let people hurt her feelings as much." "Yeah," he agreed, "she should learn to kick ass." I thanked Chuck for his idea and encouraged him to think of some ways other than fighting to help Sharlene.

I had made Sharlene's internal personality system external, and it appeared to me it was now fruitful to allow the system to internalize again, helping to strengthen the valuable aspects of a built-in support system while encouraging internal cooperation and assistance among the alters. I asked Sharlene to have an "inside meeting" with all the different parts of herself to see how many ideas they could find for how to help Sharlene not have her feelings hurt so much. Likewise, I encouraged Sharlene to have "group meetings" about whether or not they wanted to be adopted by Ann and Phillip, how they felt about Walt being in prison, and what they wanted to be when they grew up. Over time Sharlene came in and reported "We decided we want to be a therapist like you," "We decided we want Ann and Phillip to be our mother and father," and, finally, "We don't think we need to come to counseling anymore."

Sharlene's foster parents reported that her worrisome behavior had peaked during the weeks that the posttraumatic play was in high gear. Then her behavior had become more consistent, and there were fewer bouts of fluctuating behavior and forgotten statements and behaviors.

I had three or four sessions with the family to explain multiplicity, why it had developed, what it meant, and how to respond to the alters. Together, we read a book about multiplicity (Gil, 1990) to Sharlene. The parents responded very well, confirming to Sharlene that she was a good child and the grown-ups had been the ones who were bad. They clearly affirmed that they loved her and wanted her to be their special first daughter for the rest of their lives. They told her how much they loved her and how lucky they felt to have her as their daughter. The final statement of our last meeting came from Sharlene to her parents: "We love you too."

DISCUSSION

Sharlene was a victim of severe, heartless chronic abuse during her formative years. As a result of the brutal nature of the abuse, she had developed the ability to dissociate in order to mentally escape the abuse. Sharlene had developed a number of symptoms commonly associated with dissociative disorders, including forgetfulness, amnesia for the prior abuse, fluctuations in behavior, and destructive behavior to self and others.

Dissociation occurs along a continuum, with its most extreme form being a fragmentation into distinct personality types. This type of dissociation is known as multiple personality disorder (MPD) and is viewed as an adaptive response to an overwhelming reality. What is known about MPD is that it usually develops in children who endure overwhelming and extreme abuse. Usually, it is not diagnosed until adulthood, although a recent emergence of literature on the subject (Putnam, 1989; Ross, 1989) will make delayed diagnosis a less likely occurrence in the future.

The treatment of choice with individuals with multiple personalities includes verbal psychotherapy, hypnotherapy to access alters, and, eventually, an attempt to help the individual integrate the fragmented parts by encouraging co-consciousness and cooperation among the alters, internal communication, and processing of the trauma (Putnam, 1989). The other tenet of therapy seems to be the sharing of the diagnosis with the patient; Sharlene and I used her drawing of four separate alters on one page to help her understand that all her alters constituted her self.

Sharlene had fragmented enough to have two primary personalities attending the therapy. In my work with other clients with multiple personalities the alters have not been this clear-cut and available. The emergence of the alters was probably a result of the intense stress Sharlene faced on a daily basis: She had become obese and was being ridiculed and ostracized at school. Reportedly, the children at school frequently pointed at her and gathered in groups to laugh at her. This experience and the sensation of being watched penetrated Sharlene's defenses and triggered off the unconscious memory of being watched during the forced sexual activity of her early childhood.

The art work, role-playing, and accessibility to the two alters who came to therapy facilitated the treatment process for this child. However, the posttraumatic play had elements of danger in that it seemed to exacerbate the sexual arousal and resultant conditioning to abusive memories. The intervention of having the alters enter the posttraumatic play and speak directly for themselves redirected Sharlene's energy into more appropriate channels and proved to be my link between the two alters who came to treatment.

Family sessions were undertaken to discuss the multiplicity and the adoption. Fortunately, the foster parents were receptive to the notion of multiplicity as a creative survival strategy, and they were eager to learn how to respond to Sharlene and her alters. The family members pledged their love and commitment to each other during a family session after Sharlene's multiplicity was apparent; the content and timing of this session was reaffirming and beneficial to Sharlene.

Sharlene's treatment lasted 9 months. Her foster parents reported a happier, less sullen child, who made friends, joined the basketball team, and attended school more willingly. She had nightmares and periods of staying in her room alone, but overall she seemed to have greater self-confidence and communicated more freely when she felt upset.

Special Issues

COUNTERTRANSFERENCE

I have alluded to countertransference issues throughout the book but deal with them at length here to emphasize the relevance of countertransference to work with abused children. These children are extremely vulnerable, with tumultuous histories of abuse, neglect, and deprivation. Consequently, they elicit a multitude of responses from the therapist, including intense hostility, sadness, protective impulses, and/or feelings of helplessness.

During the course of therapy the child may face a variety of disappointments and stresses from such external sources as child protection services, courts, parents, foster parents, or caretakers. In particular, abused children might have to talk to police personnel and social workers, undergo physical exams, consult with district attorneys regarding court testimony, and be totally reliant on others for their future well-being.

The clinician may become invested in recommendations that are requested from authorities and may share the child's frustration and disappointment when the outcome is incompatible with expectations. On occasion, a child's plight demands special attention, and highly qualified professionals may find themselves behaving in unexpected ways. For example, one clinician treating an abused child got herself licensed as a foster parent and entered into a dual role with the child. Another clinician, whose rescuing instinct was strongly evoked, adopted a child. While these may be extremes, the clinician must carefully assess any personal conduct that threatens to develop outside the boundaries of a strict therapeutic relationship.

CLINICIAN SELF-CARE

This type of work is simultaneously rewarding and demanding. It is critical for the clinician to set limits on the number of child abuse clients seen, on the number of cases seen per day and per week, and on the number of clients accepted who have the same difficult diagnosis. For example, treating individuals with multiple personalities requires a great deal of time and effort. To build a practice limited to individuals with multiplicity would be a disservice to both clients and clinician.

Because the work is so compelling, some clinicians become literally consumed with the subject, reading only books on child abuse, attending seminars only on child abuse, and listening to hours upon hours of audiotapes on child abuse while driving.

The clinician is advised to replenish himself/herself through physical activity, vacations, and frequent changes of environment. In addition, it is important to balance the child abuse work with treatment of other, less urgent, problems. I have found balance absolutely vital to preventing burnout. I am fortunate to have the opportunity to teach, write, and do my clinical work. The rest I have learned the hard way, and I encourage every clinician to work hard on preventing burnout, which is inevitable when working in this challenging field.

CLINICIAN SAFETY

Working with abused children by necessity requires working with parents who exhibit a range of disturbing behaviors, including violence, impulsivity, and antisocial, dependent, infantilized, and histrionic personalities. The circumstances under which clinicians encounter abusive parents frequently involve coerced and involuntary contact. Therefore, some confrontations may be, at best, awkward and, at worst, dangerous.

Again, learning through trial and error, I believe clinicians working with this population should be equipped with information about handling crises. For example, it is important to meet with overtly hostile parents while another colleague is nearby. The police and district attorney should be consulted regarding obtaining restraining orders, if needed. The clinician is advised to see families with cotherapists when there is impending danger and to reserve the right to refer to another therapist if the client is threatening. In addition, the clinician may want to take self-defense classes, carry a whistle, or outfit the office with some alarm system. The clinician may also want to take some courses on working with violent people or defusing a potentially explosive situation.

Hopefully, these techniques will not become necessary, but it is best to anticipate dangerous situations rather than regret having ignored this aspect of the clinical work.

SUMMARY

The impact of child abuse and trauma can be long-term. Working with abused children provides us with a unique opportunity to help them process the painful and frightening events before the defensive mechanisms solidify in the personality, causing denial, avoidance, behavioral or play reenactments, or a variety of symptomatic behaviors.

There are few "rules" about working with abused and traumatized children; however, we can make inferences from the growing body of literature on adult survivors of abuse and other victims of trauma. The last two decades have seen an increase in interest and activity in researching the impact of childhood trauma and in determining treatment possibilities. We are now in a position to postulate treatment preferences for child victims of abuse and trauma.

The field of child therapy in general and therapy of abused children in particular is in evolution. The material contained in this book is intended to stimulate the creativity of sensitive and concerned professionals who have chosen to work with abused children and their families.

The case studies demonstrate the necessity of choosing the type of play therapy and treatment modality on a case by case basis. The child therapist must select the approaches and techniques carefully and observe the child's play actively. Children can communicate and demonstrate their hidden fears and concerns in a variety of ways. It is up to the clinician to recognize the child's attempts to communicate and to set the context for safety and learn to decode the child's words and actions. The child's medium for communication is not the spoken word. The child reveals himself/herself through play. The clinician must be patient, become fascinated by small nuances, and make purposeful choices.

The clinician must also take chances, recognizing the subtle messages from the child. The child will pace the therapy, and the therapist must respect the child's ability to go at a rate that can be tolerated.

Children who process an abusive or traumatic episode need input about the event, after their own perspective has been explored. The therapist must continue to struggle to find the perfect fit between technique and child; the prop or technique that allows the child to communicate freely.

Many traumatized children retreat into secrecy to deal with the frightening event. The clinician must make the playroom a safe sanctuary where secrecy can be shared with a trusted other. If the child avoids the work, the therapist gently but steadfastly stimulates the child's attention, providing a variety of relevant props, stories, or pictures. And once the material is being processed, the child requires assistance to feel his/her feelings, discharge them, and reorganize their perceptions of the abuse and what it means about who they were, who they are, and who they will be. Every opportunity to instill hope and a vision towards the future must be taken, so that the child feels less futile and more motivated towards growth. Every abused/traumatized child changes because of the trauma. The clinician's primary goal is to provide a reparative and corrective experience for the child.

References

Adams-Tucker, C. (1981). A socioclinical overview of 28 sex-abused children. *Child Abuse and Neglect, 5*, 361–367.

Adams-Tucker, L. (1982). Proximate effects of sexual abuse in childhood: A report on 28 children. *American Journal of Psychiatry, 139*, 1252–1256.

American Psychiatric Association (1987). *Diagnostic and statistical manual of mental disorders* (3rd ed., rev.). Washington, DC: Author.

Anthony, E. J., & Cohler, B. J. (1987). *The invulnerable child.* New York: Guilford Press.

Axline, V. M. (1964). *Dibbs in search of self.* New York: Ballantine.

Axline, V. M. (1969). *Play therapy.* New York: Ballantine.

Azar, S. T., & Wolfe, D. A. (1989). Child abuse and neglect. In E. J. Mash & R. A. Barkley (Eds.), *Treatment of childhood disorders* (pp. 451–489). New York: Guilford Press.

Barrett, M. J., Sykes, C., & Byrnes, W. (1986). A systemic model for the treatment of intrafamilial child sexual abuse. In T. S. Trapper & M. J. Barrett (Eds.), *Treating incest: A multiple systems perspective* (pp. 67–82). New York: Haworth Press.

Barrios, B. A., & O'Dell, S. L. (1989). Fears and anxieties. In E. J. Mash & R. A. Barkley (Eds.), *Treatment of childhood disorders* (pp. 167–221). New York: Guilford Press.

Beezeley, P., Martin, H. P., & Alexander, H. (1976). Comprehensive family oriented therapy. In R. E. Helfer & C. H. Kempe (Eds.), *Child abuse and neglect: The family and the community* (pp. 169–194). Cambridge, MA: Ballinger.

Bergen, M. (1958). Effect of severe trauma on a 4-year-old child. *The Psychoanalytic Study of the Child, 13,* 407–429. New York: International Universities Press.

Berliner, L., Manaois, O., & Monastersky, C. (1986). *Child sexual behavior disturbance: An assessment and treatment model.* Seattle, WA: Harborview Sexual Assault Center.

Braun, B. G. (1988). The BASK model of dissociation, *Dissociation, 1*(1), 410.

Briere, J. (1989). *Therapy for adults molested as children: Beyond survival.* New York: Springer.

Briquet, P. (1859). *Traite clinique et therapeutique de l'hysterie.* Paris: Balliere.

Burgess, A. W., Holmstrom, L. L., & McCausland, M. P. (1978). Counseling young victims and their families. In A. W. Burgess, A. N. Groth, L. L. Holmstrom, & S. M. Sgroi (Eds.), *Sexual assault of children and adolescents* (pp. 181–204). Lexington MA: Lexington Books.

Caffey, J. (1946). Multiple fractures in the long bones of infants suffering from chronic subdural hematoma. *American Journal of Roentgenology, 56,* 163–173.

Caruso, K. (1986). *Projective story-telling cards.* Redding, CA: Northwest Psychological.

Chethik, M. (1989). *Techniques of child therapy: Psychodynamic strategies.* New York: Guilford Press.

Communication Skillbuilders (1988). *Feeling cards.* Kalispel, MT: Author.

Cooper, S., & Wanerman, L. (1977). *Children in treatment: A primer for beginning psychotherapists.* New York: Brunner/Mazel.

Corder, B. F., Haizlip, T., & DeBoer, P. (1990). A pilot study for a structured, time-limited therapy group for sexually abused pre-adolescent children. *Child Abuse and Neglect, 14,* 243–251.

Courtois, C. A. (1989). *Healing the incest wound.* New York: Norton.

Davis, N. (1990). *Once upon a time....Therapeutic stories to heal abused children.* Oxon Hill, MD: Psychological Associates of Oxon Hill.

Diamond, C. B. (1988). General issues in the clinical assessment of children and adolescents. In C. J. Kestenbaum & D. T. Williams (Eds.), *Handbook of clinical assessment of children and adolescents* (Vol. 1, pp. 43–56). New York: University Press.

Dimock, P. T. (1988). Adult males sexually abused as children: Characteristics and implications for treatment. *Journal of Interpersonal Violence, 3*(2), 203–221.

Emslie, G. J., & Rosenfeld, A. (1983). Incest reported by children and adolescents hospitalized for severe psychiatric problems. *American Journal of Psychiatry, 140,* 708–711.

Erikson, E. H. (1963). *Childhood and society.* New York: Norton.

Esman, A. H. (1983). Psychoanalytic play therapy. In C. Schaefer & K. O'Connor (Eds.), *Handbook of play therapy* (pp. 11–20). New York: Wiley.

Eth, S., & Pynoos, R. S. (1985). Developmental perspective on psychic trauma in childhood, In C. R. Figley (Ed.), *Trauma and its wake* (pp. 36–52). New York: Brunner/Mazel.

Figley, C. R. (1985). *Trauma and its wake.* New York: Brunner/Mazel.

Finch, S. (1973). Adult seduction of the child: Effects on the child. *Medical Aspects of Human Sexuality, 7,* 170–187.

Finkelhor, D. (1984). *Child sexual abuse: New theory and research.* New York: The Free Press.

Finkelhor, D. (1986). *A sourcebook on child sexual abuse.* Newbury Park, CA: Sage.

Finkelhor, D., & Browne, A. (1985). The traumatic impact of child sexual abuse: A conceptualization. *American Journal of Orthopsychiatry, 55,* 530–541.

Freiberg, S. (1965). A comparison of the analytic method in two stages of child analysis. *Journal of the American Academy of Child Psychiatry, 4,* 387–400.

Freud, A. (1926). *The psychoanalytic treatment of children.* London: Imago Press.

Freud, A. (1945). Indications for child analysis. *The Psychoanalytic Study of the Child, 1,* 127–149. New York: International Universities Press.

Freud, S. (1895). Analytic Therapy. *Standard Edition, 16,* 448–463. London: Hogarth Press.

Freud, S. (1909). *Analysis of a phobia in a five-year-old boy.* London: Hogarth Press.

Friedrich, W. N. (1988). Behavior problems in sexually abused children: An adaptational perspective. In G. E. Wyatt & G. J. Powell (Eds.), *Lasting effects of child sexual abuse.* Beverly Hills, CA: Sage.

Friedrich, W. N. (1990). *Psychotherapy of sexually abused children and their families.* New York: Norton.

Friedrich, W., Berliner, L., Urquiza, A., & Beilke, R. L. (1988). Brief diagnostic group treatment of sexually abused boys. *Journal of Interpersonal Violence, 3* (3), 331–343.

Fries, M. (1937). Play technique in the analysis of young children. *Psychoanalytic Review, 24,* 233–245.

Garbarino, J., Guttman, E., & Seeley, J. W. (1986). *The psychologically battered child.* San Francisco, CA: Jossey-Bass.

Gardner, R. (1971). *Therapeutic communication with children: The mutual storytelling technique.* New York: Science House.

Giarretto, H., Giarretto, A., & Sgroi, S. (1984). Coordinated community treatment of incest. In A. W. Burgess, A. N. Groth, L. L. Holmstrom, & S. M. Sgroi (Eds.), *Sexual assault of children and adolescents* (pp. 231–240). Lexington, MA: Lexington Books.

Gil, E. (1988). *Treatment of adult survivors of childhood abuse.* Walnut Creek, CA: Launch Press.

Gil, E. (1990). *United we stand: A book for people with multiple personalities.* Walnut Creek, CA: Launch Press.

Ginott, H. G. (1961). *Group psychotherapy with children.* New York: McGraw-Hill.

Green, A. H. (1983). Dimensions of psychological trauma in abused children. *Journal of the American Association of Child Psychiatry, 22,* 231–237.

Green, A. H. (1988). The abused child and adolescent. In C. J. Kestenbaum & D. T. Williams (Eds.), *Handbook of clinical assessment of children and adolescents* (Vol. 2, pp. 842–863). New York: University Press.

Greenspan, S. I. (1981). *The clinical interview of the child.* New York: McGraw-Hill.

Groth, N. (1984). *Anatomical drawings for use in the investigation and intervention of child sexual abuse.* Dunedin, FL: Forensic Mental Health Associates.

Guerney, L. F. (1980). Client-centered (nondirective) play therapy. In C. Schaefer & K. O'Connor (Eds.), *Handbook of play therapy* (pp. 21–64). New York: Wiley.

Hambidge, G. (1955). Structured play therapy. *American Journal of Orthopsychiatry, 25,* 601–617.

Herman, J. L. (1981). *Father–daughter incest.* Cambridge, MA: Harvard University Press.

Holder, W. M. (Ed.). (1980). *Sexual abuse of children: Implications for treatment.* Denver, CO: American Humane Association.

Hunter, M. (1990). *Abused boys: The neglected victims of sexual abuse.* Lexington, MA: Lexington Books.

Itzkowitz, A. (1989). Children in placement: A place for family therapy. In L. Combrinck-Graham (Ed.), *Children in family contexts: Perspectives on treatment* (pp. 391–434). New York: Guilford Press.

James, B. (1989). *Treating traumatized children: New insights and creative interventions.* Lexington, MA: Lexington Books.

James, B., & Nasjleti, M. (1983). *Treating sexually abused children and their families.* Palo Alto, CA: Consulting Psychologist Press.

Janet, P. (1889). *L'automatisme psychologique.* Paris: Balliere.

Johnson, K. (1989). *Trauma in the lives of children.* Claremont, CA: Hunter House.

Johnson, K. (1989). *Trauma in the lives of children.* Claremont, CA: Hunter House.

Johnson-Cavanaugh, T. (1988). Child perpetrators, children who molest other children: Preliminary findings. *Child Abuse and Neglect, 12,* 219–229.

Julian, V., Mohr, C., & Lapp, J. (1980). Father–daughter incest: A descriptive analysis. In W. M. Holder (Ed.), *Sexual abuse of children: Implications for treatment.* Denver, CO: American Humane Association.

Kalff, D. (1980). *Sandplay.* Santa Monica, CA: Sigo.

Kardiner, A. (1941). *The traumatic neuroses of war.* New York: Hoeber.

Kempe, C. H., & Helfer, R. (Eds.). (1980). *The battered child* (3rd ed.). Chicago: University of Chicago Press.

Kempe, R. S., & Kempe, C. H. (1984). *The common secret: Sexual abuse of children and adolescents*. New York: Freeman.

Kent, J. T. (1980). A follow up study of abused children. In G. J. Williams & J. Money (Eds.), *Traumatic abuse and neglect of young children at home* (pp. 221–233). Baltimore, MD: Johns Hopkins University Press.

Klein, M. (1937). *The psychoanalysis of children* (2nd ed.). London: Hogarth Press.

Kluft, R. P. (1985). *Childhood antecedents of multiple personality*. Washington, DC: American Psychiatric Press.

Kraft, I. A. (1980). Group therapy with children and adolescents. In G. P. Sholevar, R. M. Benon, & B. J. Blinder (Eds.), *Emotional disorders in children and adolescents* (pp. 109–133). New York: Spectrum.

Leaman, K. M. (1980). Sexual abuse: The reactions of child and family. In K. MacFarlane, B. M. Jones, & L. L. Jenstrom (Eds.), *Sexual abuse of children: Selected readings* (DHHS Publication No. OHDS 78-30161) Washington, DC: U.S. Government Printing Office.

Levy, D. (1939). Release therapy. *American Journal of Orthopsychiatry, 9*, 713–736.

Lew, M. (1988). *Victims no longer: Men recovering from incest and other sexual child abuse*. New York: Harper & Row.

Lindemann, E. (1944). Symptomatology and management of acute grief. *American Journal of Psychiatry, 101*, 141–148.

Lindemann, E. (1944). Symptomatology and management of acute grief. *American Journal of Psychiatry, 101*, 141–148.

Long, S. (1986). Guidelines for treating young children. In K. MacFarlane, J. Waterman, S. Conerly, L. Damon, M. Durfee, & S. Long. *Sexual abuse of young children* (pp. 220–243). New York: Guilford Press.

Lusk, R., & Waterman, J. (1986). Effects of sexual abuse on children. In K. MacFarlane, J. Waterman, S. Conerly, L. Damon, M. Durfee, & S. Long (Eds.), *Sexual abuse of young children* (pp. 101–118). New York: Guilford Press.

MacFarlane, K., & Korbin, J. (1983). Confronting the incest secret long after the fact: A family study of multiple victimization with strategies for intervention. *Child Abuse and Neglect, 7*, 225–240.

MacFarlane, K., Waterman, J., Conerly, S., Damon, L., Durfee, M., & Long, S. (1986). *Sexual abuse of young children*. New York: Guilford Press.

Maclean, G. (1977). Psychic trauma and traumatic neurosis: Play therapy with a four-year-old boy. *Canadian Psychiatric Association Journal, 22*, 71–76.

MacVicar, K. (1979). Psychotherapeutic issues in the treatment of sexually abused girls. *Journal of the American Academy of Child Psychiatry, 18*, 342–353.

Mandell, J. G., Damon, L., Castaldo, P., Tauber, E., Monise, L., & Larsen, N. (1990). *Group treatment for sexually abused children*. New York: Guilford Press.

Mann, E., & McDermott, J. F. (1983). Play therapy for victims of child abuse and neglect. In C. Schaeffer & K. O'Connor (Eds.), *Handbook of play therapy* (pp. 283–307). New York: Wiley.

Martin, H. P. (1976). *The abused child.* Cambridge, MA: Ballinger.

Martin, H. P., & Rodeheffer, M. A. (1980). The psychological impact of abuse on children. In G. J. Williams & J. Money (Eds.), *Traumatic abuse and neglect of children at home* (pp. 205–212). Baltimore, MD: Johns Hopkins University Press.

Moustakas, C. (1966). *The child's discovery of himself.* New York: Ballantine.

Mrazek, P. B. (1980). Sexual abuse of children. *Journal of Child Psychology and Psychiatry and Allied Disciplines, 21,* 91–95.

MTI Film & Video (1989). *Superpuppy.* Deerfield, IL: Coronet Film & Video.

Myers, J. E. B., Bays, J., Becker, J., Berliner, L., Corwin, D. L., & Sayurtz, K. J. (1989). Expert testimony in child sexual abuse litigation. *Nebraska Law Review, 68* (1 & 2).

Nagera, H. (1980). Child psychoanalysis. In G. P. Sholevar, R. M. Benon, & B. J. Blinder (Eds.), *Emotional disorder in children and adolescents* (pp. 17–23). New York: Spectrum.

Nasjleti, M. (1980). Suffering in silence: The male incest victim. *Child Welfare, 59,* 5. New York: Child Welfare League.

Nickerson, E. T. (1973). Psychology of play and play therapy in classroom activities. *Educating Children, Spring,* 1–6.

Peterson, G. (1990). Diagnosis of childhood multiple personality disorder. *Dissociation, 3* (1), 3–9.

Piaget, J. (1969). *The mechanisms of perception.* New York: Basic Books.

Polansky, N. A., Chalmers, M. A., Williams, D. P., & Buttenwieser, E. W. (1981). *Damaged parents: An anatomy of child neglect.* Chicago: University of Chicago Press.

Polansky, N., Chalmers, M., Buttenweiser, R., & Williams, D. (1979). The isolation of the neglectful family. *American Journal of Orthopsychiatry, 49,* 149–152.

Porter, E. (1986). *Treating the young male victims of sexual assault: Issues and intervention strategies.* Syracuse, NY: Safer Society Press.

Porter, F. S., Blick, L. C., & Sgroi, S. M. (1982). Treatment of the sexually abused child. In S. Sgroi (Ed.), *Handbook of clinical intervention.* Lexington MA: Lexington Books.

Putnam, F. W. (1989). *Diagnosis and treatment of multiple personality disorder.* New York: Guilford Press.

Pynoos, R. S., & Eth, S. (1985). Developmental perspective on psychic trauma in childhood. In C. Figley (Ed.), *Trauma and its wake* (pp. 36–52). New York: Brunner/Mazel.

Radbill, S. X. (1980). Children in a world of violence: A history of child abuse. In C. H. Kempe & R. Helfer (Eds.), *The battered child* (3rd ed., pp. 3–20). Chicago: University of Chicago Press.

Reidy, T. J. (1980). The aggressive characteristics of abused and neglected children. In G. J. Williams & J. Money (Eds.), *Traumatic abuse and neglect of children at home* (pp. 213–220). Baltimore, MD: Johns Hopkins University Press.

Risin, L. I., & Koss, M. P. (1987). The sexual abuse of boys: Prevalence and descriptive characteristics of childhood victimizations. *Journal of Interpersonal Violence, 2*(3),309–323.

Rogers, C. (1951). *Client-centered therapy*. Boston: Houghton-Mifflen.

Ross, C. A. (1989). *Multiple personality disorder: Diagnosis, clinical features and treatment*. New York: Wiley.

Rothenberg, L., & Schaffer, M. (1966). The therapeutic play group: A case study. *Exceptional Children, 32*, 483–486.

Ruch, L. O., & Chandler, S. M. (1982). The crisis impact of sexual assault on three victim groups: Adult rape victims, child rape victims and incest victims. *Journal of Social Service Research, 5*, 83–100.

Rutter, B. (1978). *Only one Oliver*. Honolulu, HI: Salvation Army.

Sandler, J., Kennedy, H., & Tyson, R., (1980). *The technique of child psychoanalysis*. Cambridge, MA: Harvard University Press.

Schaefer, C. E. (1980). Play therapy. In G. P. Sholevar, R. M. Benson, & B. J. Blinder (Eds.), *Emotional disorders in children and adolescents*. New York: Spectrum.

Schaefer, C. E. (1983). Play therapy. In C. Schaefer & K. O'Connor (Eds.), *Handbook of play therapy* (pp. 95–106). New York: Wiley.

Schaefer, C. E., & O'Connor, K. J. (1983). *Handbook of play therapy*. New York: Wiley.

Scharff, D. E., & Scharff, J. S. (1987). *Object relations family therapy*, Northvale, NJ: Aronson.

Scurfield, R. M. (1985). Post-trauma stress assessment and treatment: Overview and formulations. In C. R. Figley (Ed.), *Trauma and its wake* (pp. 219–256). New York: Brunner/Mazel.

Sgroi, S. (1982). *Handbook of clinical intervention in child sexual abuse*. Lexington, MA: Lexington Books.

Sgroi, S. M., Bunk, B. S., & Wabrek, C. J. (1988). A clinical approach to adult survivors of child sexual abuse. In S. M. Sgroi (Ed.), *Vulnerable populations* (pp. 137–186). Lexington, MA: Lexington Books.

Sholevar, G. P., Benon, R. M., & Blinder, B. J. (Eds.). (1980). *Emotional disorders in children and adolescents*. New York: Spectrum.

Simari, C. G., & Baskin, D. (1982). Incestuous experiences within homosexual populations: A preliminary study. *Archives of Sexual Behavior, 11*, 329–344.

Slavson, S. R. (Ed.). (1947). *The practice of group therapy*. New York: International Universities Press.

Solomon, J. (1938). Active play therapy. *American Journal of Orthopsychiatry, 8*, 479–498.

Sours, J. A. (1980). Preschool-age children. In G. P. Sholevar, R. M. Benson, & B. J. Blinder (Eds.), *Emotional disorders in children and adolescents* (271–282). New York: Spectrum.

Summit, R. C. (1988). Hidden victims, hidden pain: Societal avoidance of child sexual abuse. In G. E. Wyatt & G. J. Powell (Eds.), *Lasting effects of child sexual abuse* (pp. 39–60). Newbury Park, CA: Sage.

Summit, R., & Kryso, J. (1978). Sexual abuse of children: A clinical spectrum. *American Journal of Orthopsychiatry, 48,* 237–251.

Terr, L. (1983). Play therapy and psychic trauma: A preliminary report. In C. E. Schaeffer & K. J. O'Connor (Eds.), *Handbook of play therapy* (pp. 308–319). New York: Wiley.

Terr, L. (1990). *Too scared to cry.* New York: Harper & Row.

Tufts New England Medical Center, Division of Child Psychiatry. (1984). *Sexually exploited children: Service and research project* (Final report for the office of Juvenile Justice and Delinquency Prevention). Washington, DC: U.S. Department of Justice.

van der Kolk, B. A. (1987). *Psychological trauma.* Washington, DC: American Psychiatric Press.

Vander Mey, B. J., & Neff, R. L. (1982). Adult-child incest: A review of research and treatment. *Adolescence, 17,* 717–735.

Wallerstein, J. S., & Kelly, J. B. (1975). The effects of parental divorce: Experiences of the preschool child. *Journal of the American Academy of Child Psychiatry, 14,* 600–616.

Waterman, J. (1986). Overview of treatment issues. In K. MacFarlane, J. Waterman, S. Conerly, L. Damon, M. Durfee, & S. Long (Eds.), *Sexual abuse of young children* (pp. 197–203). New York: Guilford Press.

White, R. W. (1966). *Lives in progress* (2nd ed.). New York: Holt, Rinehart & Winston.

Wolfe, D. A. (1987). *Child abuse implications for child development and psychopathology.* Newbury Park, CA: Sage.

Wolfenstein, M. (1965). Introduction. In M. Wolfenstein & G. Kliman (Eds.), *Children and the death of a president.* Garden City, New York: Doubleday.

Wyatt, G. E., & Powell, G. J. (Eds.). (1988). *Lasting effects of child sexual abuse.* Newbury Park, CA: Sage.

Yalom, I. D. (1975). *The theory and practice of group psychotherapy* (2nd ed.), New York: Basic Books.

Index